BORIS KRIG

FUTURE PANDEMICS

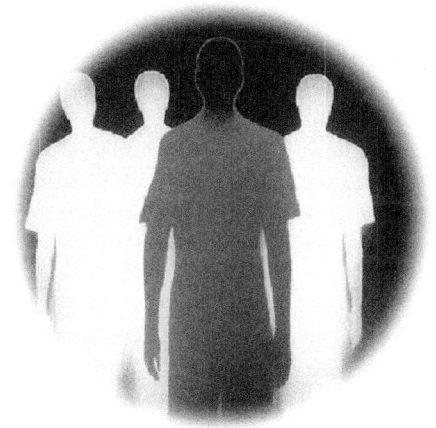

LESSONS UNLEARNED

ALTASPERA

Requests for permission to make copies of any part of this work should be e-mailed to krigerbruce@gmail.com

Published by Altaspera Publishing

Boris Kriger is a scientific writer and a versatile executive leading several companies across different industries. As a director of a clinical research organization with more than 25 years of experience, he has developed a rare blend of scientific, administrative, and leadership expertise.

He has guided multidisciplinary teams, shaped long-term strategies, and ensured rigorous compliance with FDA standards. His work spans the full cycle of clinical trials, from design and patient recruitment to data interpretation and project completion.

Future Pandemics: Lessons Unlearned

Preparing for the next pandemic means completely rethinking the medical and administrative strategies that defined the response to COVID-19. Boris Kriger, drawing on his experience as the head of a clinical research center, he argues that the world's obsession with vaccines—while valuable—came at the cost of neglecting the urgent development of drugs that could directly suppress viral replication. Instead of focusing solely on prevention, he insists, we must invest in treatments that can swiftly weaken a virus once it has entered the body, reducing both the severity and duration of illness.

The book explores the role of modern technology in this new vision of preparedness. Artificial intelligence, the author explains, can be harnessed to analyze vast amounts of medical data, identify emerging patterns of infection, and accelerate the discovery of effective therapeutics. Telemedicine, too, has proven its worth—allowing doctors to diagnose and monitor patients from afar, minimizing the risk of contagion while keeping healthcare accessible. Even drones find a place in this futuristic strategy: deployed to deliver medicines and supplies to remote or quarantine areas without any human contact, they transform logistics into a shield against transmission.

In short, the author's message is clear: if we are to survive the next great pandemic, we must stop trying to return to "normal." Instead, we must build a smarter, more adaptive world—one that treats preparedness not as panic after the fact, but as a permanent and deliberate state of readiness.

Keywords

Pandemics, COVID, Decentralization, Artificial Intelligence, Telemedicine, Preparedness, Autonomous Living

Contents

INTRODUCTION

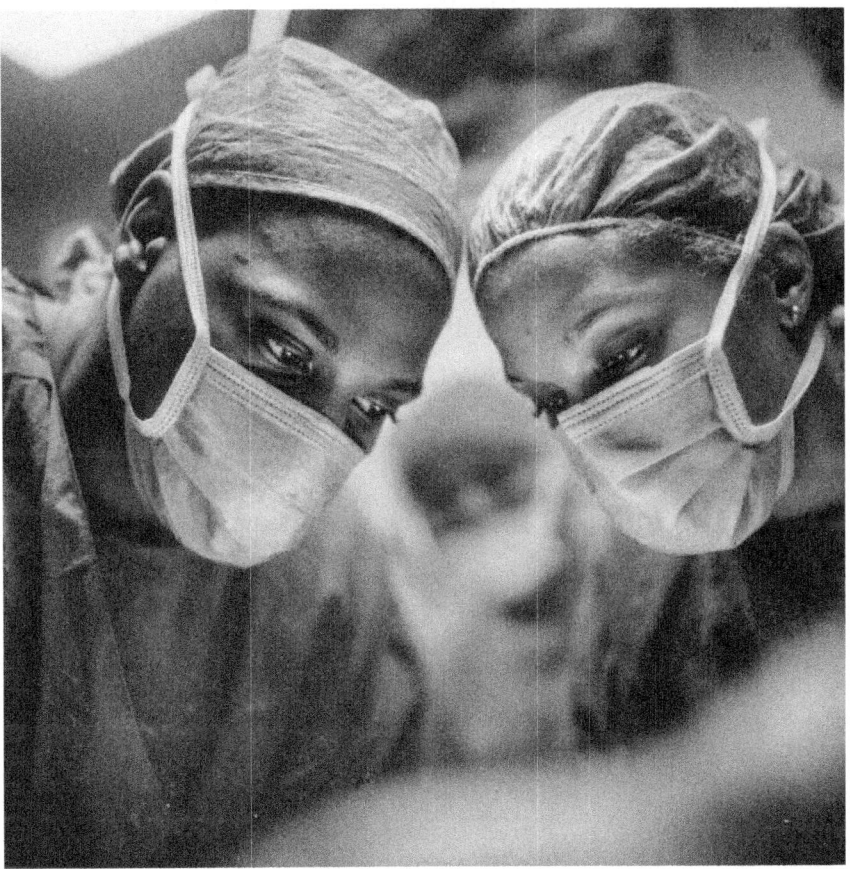

The last pandemic did not defeat science. It defeated systems. The distinction is essential. Science, as a human endeavor, performed as it always has—messy, self-correcting, brilliant in bursts, confused in others, but fundamentally sound. What failed, catastrophically and repeatedly, were the systems built to translate scientific knowledge into collective action. This book is not an indictment of the individuals who labored under impossible conditions—scientists, doctors, nurses, public health workers, and civil servants who gave their best while the machinery they depended on sputtered, jammed, or collapsed outright. It is, instead, a critique of that machinery itself: the institutions, hierarchies, and bureaucratic reflexes that turned a global health crisis into a systemic debacle.

We are accustomed to thinking of pandemics as tests of biology, but they are also tests of design—organizational, informational, and moral design. When those systems fail, the virus becomes only one of the pathogens at work. The other is institutional inertia. What spread across borders faster than any variant of the virus was confusion: governments contradicting their own experts, data systems unable to talk to one another, supply chains disintegrating under their own complexity, and entire nations improvising policy on the fly while insisting on the illusion of control.

Science itself was not silent or absent. Laboratories sequenced genomes in record time. Epidemiologists mapped contagion patterns within weeks. Vaccines, once the stuff of decade-long projects, arrived in under a year. But information and capability do not equal coherence. Knowledge without coordination is noise, and noise was what much of the world heard—shouting from podiums, scrolling numbers of cases and deaths, contradictory orders that changed with each new headline. The deeper failure lay in the inability to integrate knowledge into governance, and governance into trust.

What makes this failure systemic rather than personal is that no single decision, and no single leader, explains it. The pattern repeated across borders and political ideologies. It was not the fault of one country's arrogance or another's complacency, but of a shared architecture of modern institutions—fragmented, risk-averse, allergic to transparency, and calibrated for stability rather than agility. The systems built to prevent disaster proved too brittle to adapt when disaster arrived in a form they had not rehearsed.

The aim here is not to assign blame, but to understand the anatomy of that brittleness. Why did so many agencies built for crisis management move slower than the crises they were meant to manage? Why did communication systems designed for accuracy become engines of misinformation? Why did structures meant to protect the public often act instead to protect themselves—from accountability, from uncertainty, from change?

This book argues that the great failure of the pandemic was not a failure of knowledge but of translation—between science and policy, between expertise and decision, between data and meaning. The pandemic revealed that our institutions, for all their sophistication, remain bound to industrial-age habits of control and secrecy in a networked, real-time world. They were designed for linear problems, not cascading ones. For stability, not turbulence. For authority, not adaptation.

If this sounds harsh, it is because systems—unlike people—do not deserve sympathy. They deserve scrutiny. The scientists who raised alarms early, the public health workers who improvised solutions in underfunded departments, the local officials who made decisions with incomplete data—these are not the culprits of this story. They are its witnesses and, too often, its casualties.

The pandemic was not merely a biological event but a mirror, reflecting the architecture of the societies it struck. What it showed us was not new: the fragility of global cooperation, the politicization of expertise, the commodification of health. But it showed them with such clarity that we could no longer pretend not to see. This book begins from that uncomfortable clarity—not to mourn what failed, but to understand why, and how it might be rebuilt before the next inevitable test.

The failure was not of science. It was of the systems meant to carry science into the world—and the world's failure to carry those systems forward when they mattered most.

The central argument of this book rests on a simple but neglected truth: vaccines and antivirals are not rivals. They are partners in a complete public health defense. To frame them as competitors is to misunderstand the nature of the threat we faced—and will face again. The pandemic revealed how deeply our institutions have internalized the idea that prevention and treatment exist on opposite sides of a binary, when in reality they form a continuum. Vaccines guard the gates; antivirals fight within the walls. Both are indispensable, and both depend on systems capable of delivering them swiftly and fairly.

Much of the early pandemic response revolved, understandably, around vaccines. They offered the promise of control, of an end. But the singular fixation on vaccination as the sole path to safety blinded many institutions to an equally vital weapon: rapid, accessible treatment. Vaccines protect populations; antivirals protect individuals. When used together, they prevent the collapse of both bodies and systems. To rely on one without the other is like defending a city with walls but no medics, or medics but no walls.

The story of Paxlovid—and of other antiviral treatments like it—is not one of scientific discovery alone, but of strategic neglect. These medicines were available, effective, and underused. They could have reduced deaths, eased the pressure on hospitals, and, perhaps most importantly, tempered the pervasive sense of helplessness that fueled both panic and political dysfunction. Yet deployment lagged behind need, mired in bureaucracy, confusion, and an institutional culture that equated early treatment with defeat.

Early treatment is not an admission of failure. It is a form of preparedness. Every infection prevented is a victory; every infection treated swiftly is another. A resilient system recognizes both. The capacity to test and treat early—within days, not weeks—is not merely a medical asset but a psychological one. It reassures citizens that infection is not a sentence, that the state is not powerless, and that the tools of science exist to protect rather than scold them. When people believe there are effective options beyond isolation and fear, social cohesion strengthens. The opposite—messaging that oscillates between denial and despair—breeds distrust, conspiracy, and fatigue.

Antivirals like Paxlovid represent more than pharmaceutical success; they embody a philosophy of response. They bridge the gap between prevention and care, between population-level policy and personal agency. In a world where pandemics move faster than bureaucracies, a system that can distribute treatment as nimbly as it delivers information becomes the difference between control and chaos.

To argue for antivirals is not to diminish vaccines. It is to complete the circle that vaccines alone cannot close. Vaccination campaigns, no matter how successful, will always leave gaps—people unvaccinated, immunity waning, new variants emerging. Antivirals are the fail-safe, the second layer that catches what prevention cannot. Together, they create not a perfect shield, but a resilient one.

The lesson is clear: strategy must evolve from a singular obsession with stopping transmission to a more balanced architecture—prevent, detect, treat. That third pillar has too often been treated as an afterthought. It must instead become a foundation. In future pandemics, the measure of preparedness will not be how fast we can build a vaccine, but how seamlessly we can pair that vaccine with early, equitable access to treatment.

This book defends that position unapologetically. It is not a manifesto for miracle drugs, nor a dismissal of the extraordinary achievement of global vaccination. It is a call to design systems that do not force false choices between prevention and response, between science and logistics, between hope and realism. For in the end, what failed was not the medicine—but our ability to deliver it in time.

If the pandemic revealed anything beyond our medical vulnerability, it was the disarray of our information. Data—the lifeblood of any modern response—was scattered across incompatible systems, trapped in bureaucratic silos, and guarded more fiercely than it was shared. Hospitals, laboratories, local governments, and federal agencies each spoke their own dialect of statistics, often incomprehensible to one another. The result was paralysis disguised as precision: numbers everywhere, coherence nowhere. To rebuild a resilient public health system, we must begin by rebuilding the way it knows itself.

This book argues for the creation of a unified national health-data infrastructure—a network capable of gathering, analyzing, and communicating health information in real time, securely and intelligently. Such a proposal inevitably raises fears: surveillance, loss of privacy, government overreach. These are not paranoid anxieties; they are legitimate concerns rooted in history and experience. But acknowledging them must not mean surrendering to them. The choice is not between safety and privacy, but between chaos and accountability. The key lies in design.

A well-designed system does not treat privacy as an afterthought; it builds it into its architecture. Transparency, encryption, and multilayer oversight can ensure that data serves the public without betraying the individual. The principle is simple: no one person, agency, or corporation should ever hold unchecked power over information. Access must be distributed, purposes strictly defined, and all activity subject to independent audit. Encryption and anonymization should be default settings, not optional upgrades. And transparency—

publishing what data is collected, how it is used, and by whom—should be the system's oxygen, not its threat.

The absence of such an infrastructure during the pandemic was not a triumph of privacy; it was a catastrophe of fragmentation. Lives were lost not because data was hoarded maliciously, but because it was scattered incompetently. Local officials could not see national trends; national planners could not detect local surges; hospitals competed for supplies without visibility into collective need. The irony is that the lack of shared information made everyone more vulnerable, not less. Protecting privacy by preventing connection is like protecting property by refusing to build roads.

A unified health-data network, properly governed, can make privacy stronger by making responsibility traceable. When data flows through transparent, encrypted systems rather than opaque back channels, abuses are easier to detect and harder to conceal. Every access, every query, every algorithmic decision can be logged, reviewed, and justified. The current patchwork, by contrast, hides incompetence as easily as it hides intrusion. Fragmentation breeds both inefficiency and impunity.

Privacy, then, must not be seen as a fortress but as a framework—a living contract between citizens and their institutions. The contract's legitimacy depends on trust, and trust depends on visibility. The pandemic made clear that public trust cannot be maintained by secrecy. It must be earned through consistent honesty about what the system is doing and why. If the public can see the structure of oversight—independent boards, ethical review panels, data-use charters—they are more likely to grant consent to the collective use of their information.

The goal is not a national database of citizens' health histories, but a national nervous system for public health—responsive, secure, and adaptive. Such a system could detect outbreaks early, target resources intelligently, and coordinate responses without the confusion that cost so much time and credibility during the last crisis. It could empower local authorities with real-time insights rather than outdated spreadsheets, and it could give citizens confidence that their data serves a shared purpose rather than an invisible one.

The pandemic showed that ignorance can be just as dangerous as intrusion. Data without protection is perilous, but so is protection without data. Between those extremes lies the space where intelligent systems and ethical design can coexist. This book argues that we must inhabit that space—open-eyed, technologically capable, and morally vigilant—if we are to transform the next pandemic from a tragedy of blindness into a triumph of preparedness.

Among the most striking lessons of the pandemic was the collapse of proximity. Medicine, once built on the intimacy of touch and presence, was forced to migrate into the digital ether almost overnight. Waiting rooms emptied, hospitals became fortresses, and screens became lifelines. Telemedicine, once an experiment in convenience, suddenly became the backbone of survival. And alongside it, algorithms—those tireless pattern-recognizers we alternately fear and overpraise—emerged as the only way to extend medical judgment to the scale the crisis demanded.

This book does not idealize these tools. Telemedicine and AI diagnostics are imperfect, limited, and deeply dependent on human oversight. Algorithms are not doctors, and screens cannot replace hands. Yet in a moment when need outstripped capacity by orders of magnitude, perfection was not an option. The alternative to scalable technology was not better care, but no care at all. The moral question was not whether machines could equal human judgment, but whether they could amplify it fast enough to save lives that otherwise would not be reached in time.

The myth of medical perfection—the belief that every diagnosis must be certain, every consultation personal, every decision unanimous—proved incompatible with the realities of crisis. When systems are overwhelmed, medicine becomes triage. The art of triage is not precision; it is prioritization. It is the disciplined, compassionate act of doing the most good for the most people with the tools available. In that sense, AI and telemedicine were not technological shortcuts but moral instruments: ways to scale empathy when proximity was impossible.

Telemedicine democratized access in an hour of lockdowns. Patients who might otherwise have gone unseen—because of geography, fear, or contagion—could reach clinicians through screens. AI systems, trained on vast medical datasets, helped flag early warning signs, identify high-risk patients, and suggest courses of action where specialists were scarce. These systems did not replace expertise; they multiplied its reach. And while their predictions were sometimes flawed, they were at least consistent—immune to fatigue, distraction, and despair.

Critics rightly warn that algorithms inherit biases from the data that shapes them. That is true—and dangerous. A biased model can encode injustice at the speed of computation. But inaction, too, is a bias: a bias toward the status quo, toward scarcity and paralysis. The challenge, therefore, is not whether to use AI in health crises, but how to use it ethically—openly, audibly, and under rigorous supervision. A transparent algorithm can be audited and improved; an overburdened human system cannot.

When used properly, these technologies do not strip medicine of humanity—they restore it, by freeing clinicians from the impossible expectation of omnipresence. AI does not think for doctors; it helps them see patterns too large for any one mind. Telemedicine does not replace the human encounter; it extends it beyond walls and time zones. Together, they form the nervous system of a modern health response—elastic, adaptive, and capable of holding the line when the physical infrastructure falters.

The pandemic exposed the limits of every traditional boundary in healthcare: between hospitals and homes, between doctors and patients, between expertise and accessibility. Technology blurred those boundaries out of necessity. The next crisis will demand that we make that blurring deliberate. A resilient system must be able to pivot instantly from centralized to distributed care, from manual to augmented judgment, from physical to virtual presence—without sacrificing trust or ethics in the process.

Acknowledging the limitations of telemedicine and AI is not an argument against them. It is an argument for realism. In moments of systemic overload, the choice is never between ideal and flawed—it is between scalable triage and catastrophic neglect. Algorithms will err; networks will fail; connections will drop. But a system that refuses to use them because they are imperfect risks far greater imperfection: a void. The goal, therefore, is not to worship technology, but to integrate it with humility—using its reach to preserve what is most irreplaceable in medicine: human judgment, compassion, and the will to act even when certainty is impossible.

During the pandemic, the world discovered that logistics—not medicine—often determined survival. Vaccines, tests, masks, and medicines were developed at astonishing speed, yet they too often sat in warehouses, or expired in transit, or arrived months too late to matter. Trucks stalled in traffic, supply chains buckled under their own complexity, and rural communities watched drones deliver packages of consumer goods while medical supplies waited for the next available driver. The bottleneck was not innovation, but distribution. The ability to move critical resources safely, quickly, and efficiently proved as decisive as the ability to invent them.

This book argues that drone-based logistics and autonomous delivery systems are not science fiction; they are overdue infrastructure. They represent a shift from reactive transport to anticipatory mobility—networks that can deliver vital goods precisely where and when they are needed, without risking human couriers or relying on brittle supply lines. The technology exists; the challenge is the courage to deploy it at scale.

Skeptics often dismiss the idea of autonomous delivery as impractical, costly, or untested. In truth, the opposite is already being proven. Long before the pandemic, pilot programs were underway in countries across the world. In Rwanda and Ghana, drones operated by companies like Zipline have delivered blood, vaccines, and emergency medicines to remote clinics for years—saving lives and demonstrating reliability under rugged conditions. In the United States, pilot projects run by logistics giants, universities, and emergency-response agencies have shown that drones can deliver small payloads safely across urban, suburban, and rural airspace. Autonomous ground vehicles, too, have been tested for contactless delivery in dense cityscapes. These are not prototypes in search of purpose; they are proven systems awaiting political and institutional permission to grow.

Feasibility, then, is no longer the question. The real obstacle is inertia—the bureaucratic gravity of outdated models of distribution. Public health systems continue to rely on 20th-century logistics: centralized warehouses, paper manifests, and manual routing that collapses under the weight of sudden demand. The cost of this stagnation is invisible until the crisis hits, at which point it becomes catastrophic. Every hour lost to logistics during an outbreak translates into hospitalizations that could have been prevented and lives that could have been saved.

Modernizing distribution is not a luxury; it is preparedness. Drones can reach quarantine zones, deliver medicines to patients isolating at home, transport samples to laboratories faster than road traffic, and maintain operations when weather or infrastructure fail. In emergencies, where every minute counts, autonomy buys time—and time is the currency of survival. The argument is not that drones or robots will replace human logistics, but that they will augment it, creating a layered, resilient network that continues functioning even when traditional channels break down.

Cost, often cited as a barrier, must be measured against the cost of failure. The economic and human losses from supply-chain collapse during the pandemic dwarf any investment required to automate and modernize distribution. The expense of inaction is not theoretical; it has already been paid in lost productivity, preventable deaths, and shattered trust. By contrast, autonomous delivery offers compounding returns: faster response times, lower operational costs, and reduced dependency on strained human labor during crises.

Critics warn that technology can dehumanize response systems, but there is nothing humane about a logistics model that cannot deliver care to those who need it most. Drones and autonomous vehicles are not symbols of cold automation; they are instruments of access. They make equity logistically possible—extending the reach of health systems into the very geographies that have historically been left behind.

The future of crisis response will not be defined only by how we make medicine, but by how we move it. A modernized, drone-enabled logistics network is not a futuristic add-on; it is a strategic necessity. It converts speed into safety, geography into opportunity, and distance into solvable engineering rather than fatal inevitability. The pandemic taught us that distribution is destiny. The next one will test whether we learned it.

The book does not argue that technology eliminates human irrationality; rather, it argues that technology eliminates the layers of preventable risk that arise precisely because humans are irrational. Automation has already transformed safety and reliability across aviation, manufacturing, energy systems, medicine, and transportation. Nowhere has automation made humans wiser or calmer; it has simply reduced the number of situations in which human panic, fatigue, bias, or inconsistency can cause harm. This is not technological determinism. It is a sober recognition of empirical fact: when systems automate what humans routinely mishandle, outcomes become dramatically safer. Preparedness is not the belief that technology replaces humanity, but the insistence that we no longer leave civilization-level vulnerabilities in the hands of creatures who evolved to flee lions, not to coordinate supply chains.

The argument that "algorithms may fail" misunderstands what they are being compared to. Algorithms do not need to be perfect; they only need to be better than the chaos, inconsistency, and emotional volatility that human decision-making repeatedly demonstrates. Machines do not panic, stall, lie, hide data, protect political interests, retaliate against colleagues, misplace shipments, or change protocols out of fear or vanity. Their errors are systematic and therefore correctable, while human errors are erratic and often catastrophic. In every domain where outcomes depend on precision, speed, and consistency, even imperfect algorithms outperform the most well-intentioned committees. The question, therefore, is not whether machines might make mistakes, but why we continue to entrust life-critical systems to a species that has proven, time and again, that it cannot coordinate itself under pressure.

The pandemic turned cities—the triumphs of human concentration—into symbols of vulnerability. The very density that made them efficient and creative also made them fragile. Within weeks, once-vibrant centers of commerce and culture became epidemiological accelerants: subways as arteries of contagion, apartment towers as echo chambers of isolation, office districts as ghost zones. For a moment, the centuries-old equation of "urban equals progress" appeared inverted. But to suggest that cities are obsolete is to misunderstand the lesson. What failed was not the idea of cities, but the assumption that they must remain our only viable pattern of life.

This book argues for a concept of *urban dispersal* and *modular housing* not as a retreat from modernity, but as an evolution of it—a diversification strategy for human settlement in an age of recurring shocks. The goal is not to abandon the metropolis, but to relieve it; not to dismantle density, but to make it optional. True resilience lies in choice: the ability of societies to adapt living patterns without economic or social collapse when one structure becomes unsafe, overloaded, or uninhabitable.

Urban dispersal does not mean isolation. It means designing systems in which work, education, healthcare, and culture can flourish beyond the gravitational pull of megacities. The pandemic proved that digital infrastructure can decentralize productivity as effectively as highways once centralized it. When remote work, telemedicine, and autonomous logistics become permanent capabilities, the necessity of forcing millions into the same few urban cores begins to fade. A distributed model of living—supported by technology and connected by resilient networks—offers the same access to opportunity without the same exposure to systemic failure.

Modular housing is the architectural counterpart of that idea: flexible, rapidly deployable, and adaptable to changing conditions. Unlike the static towers and sprawling suburbs of the industrial era, modular housing can expand, contract, relocate, and reconfigure. It is architecture as infrastructure—designed for speed, safety, and adaptability. In a crisis, modular units can become temporary shelters or field clinics; in peacetime, they can evolve into permanent neighborhoods. This is not utopian futurism. It is a pragmatic response to a century in which mobility and climate, migration and health, will repeatedly test our ability to live well in flux.

Critics often misread dispersal strategies as anti-city romanticism, as though the argument were to trade skyscrapers for cabins. But the real proposal is diversification: building a spectrum of living environments rather than a monoculture of dependence on dense hubs. Just as biodiversity protects an ecosystem, variety in human settlement protects a civilization. A country of only cities is as brittle as a forest of a single species. When one fails, the entire system burns.

The vision here is not pastoral nostalgia but systemic flexibility. Imagine a network of smaller, well-connected communities—each equipped with reliable broadband, renewable energy, modular healthcare facilities, and autonomous supply chains. People would not be *exiled* from cities, but *freed* from their necessity. Density would become a choice, not an economic trap. In crises—whether viral, environmental, or infrastructural—population could redistribute temporarily without chaos, because the architecture of life outside the metropolis would already exist.

The cost of inaction, as always, is visible in hindsight. When cities became unsafe, millions tried to flee, only to find nowhere ready to receive them. Housing markets warped, rural systems buckled, and governments scrambled to improvise relocation measures that should have been designed decades earlier. The next crisis—pandemic, climate, or cyber—will likely test the same weak points. The question is not whether people *can* live differently, but whether our systems will allow them to without penalty.

Urban dispersal and modular housing offer a blueprint for resilience that transcends emergency. They decentralize risk, democratize opportunity, and turn geography into a variable rather than a vulnerability. This is not anti-urban idealism; it is twenty-first-century realism. The great cities will endure—they always do—but the next measure of progress will not be how tall our skylines grow, but how flexibly our societies can breathe when the air within them grows dangerous.

The pandemic was not just a biological crisis—it was an information crisis, a political crisis, and a crisis of trust. The virus moved invisibly through populations, but misinformation moved faster still, amplified by political theatrics and the machinery of spectacle that modern governance has become. Leaders across the world—left, right, authoritarian, democratic—found themselves not merely fighting a pathogen but performing against it, often mistaking public communication for public health. Yet this book does not seek to condemn individuals or parties. It seeks to diagnose a system-wide disorder: the conversion of governance into theater, and information into noise.

This is not a partisan critique. It is not a tally of which country, ideology, or administration failed the most. The failure was universal, transcending ideology and geography. Governments of every political stripe—progressive and conservative, centralized and federal, technocratic and populist—succumbed to the same pattern of confusion: inconsistent messaging, reactive policies, and the substitution of narrative management for problem-solving. The cause was not malice but structure—a communication system built for control, not for clarity.

In times of peace, politics thrives on spectacle: slogans, rivalries, announcements crafted for cameras rather than outcomes. But pandemics are the opposite of theater. They demand precision, humility, and consistency—the very qualities that political ecosystems, trained for perpetual campaigning, often suppress. When the crisis struck, those instincts did not vanish; they metastasized. Press conferences became performances of certainty in a world of uncertainty. Every statement was filtered through the calculus of optics. The result was chaos disguised as competence—officials contradicting scientists, scientists censored by officials, and citizens trapped in the resulting fog of mistrust.

The critique here is structural. Modern governments, for all their intelligence and technology, communicate through systems designed for an earlier era of information scarcity. Those systems break under the pressure of digital abundance. Messages intended to reassure the public are distorted by algorithmic incentives, weaponized by bad actors, and diluted by sheer volume. The more governments tried to control the narrative, the less credible they became. The vacuum that followed was filled by rumor, speculation, and rage.

To understand this is not to vilify leaders, but to recognize the architecture of failure. The machinery of political communication—press offices, social media strategies, bureaucratic approval chains—proved too slow and too filtered to adapt. In an environment that demanded agile truth-telling, institutions defaulted to defensive messaging. The instinct to appear composed outweighed the need to be transparent. Yet uncertainty, when hidden, grows into panic. Honesty, when delayed, sounds like retreat.

This is why the book speaks not of partisan mismanagement but of systemic misalignment. The global response faltered because the very channels through which governments connect with citizens have become entangled with the incentives of performance—poll numbers, media cycles, outrage economies. The communications infrastructure of democracy, and of many autocracies alike, has been rewired for attention rather than comprehension. In a pandemic, attention kills.

The solution is not to silence politics but to re-engineer its voice. Public communication must evolve from theater to transmission—from curated image to functional literacy. That means admitting uncertainty when it exists, empowering technical experts to speak without censorship, and designing platforms where clarity is rewarded more than virality. Trust cannot be legislated or tweeted into existence; it must be earned through systems that make honesty operational rather than optional.

This book is written in that spirit of reform, not accusation. It recognizes that politicians, too, are trapped in the machinery they inherited—systems that penalize humility, reward performance, and measure success by the minute hand of public opinion. The pandemic merely exposed those weaknesses in their rawest form. The goal here is not to blame, but to illuminate the architecture of failure so that it can be rebuilt.

What we witnessed was not the collapse of governance, but of communication. Governments did not stop functioning; they stopped being believed. Restoring that belief—through structural transparency, institutional honesty, and the depoliticization of truth—is the work ahead. The lesson is not that one party, leader, or nation failed more than others. It is that the stage itself must be redesigned if we are to stop mistaking applause for understanding, and headlines for health.

Every great crisis reveals what a civilization values most—and what it misunderstands most deeply. During the pandemic, the world responded not only with science and policy, but with story. We told ourselves tales of heroism and sacrifice, of villains and incompetence, of redemption through endurance. These narratives helped us make sense of chaos, but they also obscured the machinery of response. They turned a logistical emergency into a moral drama. And while we argued about virtue, the systems that actually determined life and death—supply chains, data networks, hospitals, coordination protocols—buckled under neglect.

This book insists on a shift in perspective: pandemics are not wars to be won by courage, nor moral reckonings to be resolved by judgment. They are infrastructure problems—complex, mechanical, and solvable through design. The virus did not respond to speeches, to patriotism, or to outrage. It responded to velocity, to logistics, to timing. Where systems were prepared, people lived. Where they were not, no amount of heroism could compensate.

This is not to diminish the courage of doctors, nurses, scientists, and essential workers. Their labor sustained civilization when systems failed them. But courage, however noble, is not a substitute for architecture. A society that relies on heroism has already admitted to structural failure. Heroes emerge when systems collapse; engineers prevent the collapse altogether. The goal, therefore, is not to inspire more self-sacrifice, but to build systems that do not require it.

Emotional narratives—panic, blame, triumph—are comforting because they are human-scale. They give faces to suffering, names to villains, arcs to chaos. But pandemics operate at scales beyond individual morality. They are governed by logistics, not sentiment. A mask shortage is not a tragedy of character; it is a failure of procurement. A delay in test results is not a story of bureaucratic apathy; it is a data infrastructure bottleneck. When we frame these failures as moral instead of mechanical, we prevent ourselves from fixing them.

The pandemic revealed how deeply our institutions are shaped by emotion disguised as principle. Policies were announced to *signal* control rather than achieve it. Leaders equated urgency with drama, empathy with improvisation. Every press conference became an episode in a global morality play, complete with heroes, villains, and applause lines. Meanwhile, the quiet work of logistics—the design of distribution routes, the modeling of hospital capacity, the management of cold chains—remained underfunded, unglamorous, and invisible. Yet it was in those hidden details, not in the televised declarations, that outcomes were decided.

The argument here is not against empathy or communication, but against the illusion that emotion is action. Outrage is not coordination. Gratitude is not preparedness. To truly honor the heroism we witnessed, we must build systems that make such heroism unnecessary. The next pandemic will not be defeated by moral fervor, but by engineering—by the disciplined, often boring work of constructing redundancy, mapping supply chains, simulating failures, and rehearsing the impossible until it becomes routine.

Treating pandemics as infrastructure problems means designing for inevitability rather than improvising for catastrophe. It means accepting that resilience is measurable not in headlines but in throughput—in how quickly information moves, how predictably supplies arrive, how seamlessly institutions communicate. These are not moral questions; they are design questions. But as long as politics rewards emotional performance over technical competence, we will continue to respond to systemic crises with cinematic gestures instead of structural reform.

This book proposes that we reframe preparedness as an engineering discipline, not a crusade. The pandemic was not a test of collective virtue; it was a stress test of collective systems. And those systems, not the people within them, were found wanting. The lesson is not to be braver next time, but to be better built. Because viruses do not care about our courage. They care only about our capacity to deliver oxygen, medicine, and data on time.

When we stop moralizing our failures, we can finally start fixing them.

Hospitals are the cathedrals of modern medicine—vast, intricate, indispensable. Within their walls, the miracles of contemporary care unfold every day: organ transplants, trauma surgery, intensive therapies. Yet the pandemic revealed a truth that our health systems have long resisted: these cathedrals, magnificent as they are, cannot stand alone. They are the heart of healthcare, but a heart without a circulatory system cannot sustain life. When crisis strikes, centralized hospitals—by design—become bottlenecks. Their strength is specialization, but their weakness is rigidity. When patients arrive faster than the system can process them, even the best hospitals become monuments to paralysis.

This book argues that resilience requires not just great hospitals, but distributed capacity—rapid, mobile, modular units that extend the reach of medicine far beyond the walls of permanent institutions. Centralized care must remain the anchor, but it cannot be the only line of defense. In a pandemic, disaster, or mass casualty event, the ability to scale care outward—to bring diagnosis, treatment, and stabilization closer to where people actually are—is the difference between a system under strain and a system in collapse.

During the pandemic, hospitals across the world became symbols of both heroism and limitation. Images of overrun emergency rooms, improvised corridors of stretchers, and exhausted staff were not failures of medicine but of logistics. Beds were not the only shortage—oxygen, ventilators, and personnel were trapped in rigid supply chains, unable to flow where the need shifted daily. Centralization amplified vulnerability. The closer a system is to its capacity limit, the less margin it has to adapt. Distributed care, by contrast, introduces elasticity. Mobile units can move, expand, and contract; they transform a static system into a dynamic one.

This concept is not theoretical. It has precedents in humanitarian medicine, disaster response, and military logistics. Field hospitals and mobile triage units have long demonstrated that high-quality care can be delivered in modular, rapidly deployable formats. Technology now makes it possible to elevate those models from emergency improvisation to standing infrastructure: self-contained clinics powered by renewable energy, equipped with telemedicine links, autonomous supply delivery, and diagnostic AI. In normal times, such units can serve rural or underserved populations; in crises, they can surge into hotspots within hours, stabilizing patients before hospitals overflow.

To advocate for distributed care is not to diminish the role of centralized hospitals, but to protect them. The best way to keep hospitals functional is to ensure they are not asked to do everything at once. By decentralizing the first stages of diagnosis and stabilization—testing, early treatment, routine monitoring—we reserve hospital capacity for the complex and critical. The system becomes layered rather than linear, flexible rather than fragile.

This approach also redefines what preparedness looks like. Stockpiling supplies is necessary but insufficient. We must also stockpile *mobility*: vehicles, tents, modular units, trained teams that can assemble into functioning clinics within days. These are not just physical assets but organizational muscles, honed by rehearsal and ready for activation. The cost of building them is far lower than the cost of letting hospitals drown under preventable load.

Some critics imagine that mobile care implies lower standards—that what moves must be makeshift. In reality, distributed systems can uphold the same clinical standards as fixed hospitals, precisely because technology has shrunk the footprint of diagnosis and monitoring. Portable imaging, point-of-care testing, digital records, and teleconsultation can turn a parking lot into a functioning ward. The barrier is not capability but imagination—and, often, regulation.

What the pandemic taught us is that no single institution, however advanced, can absorb a systemic shock alone. The next crisis will not be defeated by bigger hospitals, but by smarter networks—networks that understand care as something that flows rather than gathers. Centralized hospitals will always remain the irreplaceable hubs of expertise and complexity. But around them, we must build a constellation of mobile, adaptive nodes that can catch the overflow before it becomes tragedy.

Distributed capacity is not redundancy; it is resilience. It ensures that care is not a place but a system—one that expands under pressure instead of breaking. In the world ahead, where crises will be faster, larger, and more intertwined, our health systems must learn to behave like living organisms: flexible, responsive, capable of rerouting resources in real time. The age of immovable infrastructure is ending. The age of adaptable care must begin.

The argument at the heart of this book is that technological readiness—the capacity to prevent, contain, and mitigate catastrophe through foresight and design—is not a luxury of advanced societies but the moral floor of any responsible one. Civilization, properly understood, is not measured by its monuments or markets, but by how it anticipates suffering before it arrives. A society that learns only through failure is not resilient; it is negligent.

To treat preparedness as a form of utopian futurism is to mistake competence for fantasy. We have lived too long under the illusion that technology is something that happens to us, not something we are responsible for. The pandemic shattered that illusion. The tools we needed—data integration, rapid testing, remote diagnostics, antiviral distribution—were within reach, and often already invented. What was missing was not innovation but deployment: the unglamorous work of connecting the possible to the practical. The failure to do so was not technological—it was moral.

Preparedness is the pragmatism of empathy. It recognizes that the truest compassion is not reactive but preventive—that the highest form of care is to reduce the number of people who will need to be cared for later. A vaccine factory that can pivot to new pathogens in weeks; a logistics network that can deliver oxygen to remote towns before shortages turn lethal; a health-data system that can see outbreaks forming in real time—these are not dreams of a distant future. They are the baseline expectations of a society that takes its citizens' lives seriously.

This book's defense of technological readiness does not stem from faith in machines, but from realism about human limits. We are brilliant in moments of crisis and lazy in stretches of calm. We mistake survival for success and improvise heroically where we should have engineered soberly. Preparedness is the discipline that prevents that cycle—the deliberate choice to invest in systems before disaster makes them mandatory. It is not an act of fear, but of maturity.

Critics often cast technological ambition as hubris: a desire to dominate nature or insulate ourselves from risk. Yet true preparedness is humility in action. It begins with the admission that the future will test us, that chaos is certain, and that no amount of rhetoric will stop the next virus, fire, or flood. To prepare is not to play god; it is to acknowledge that we are fragile, interdependent creatures in need of good tools. It is the moral duty of a civilization to build those tools—not because they guarantee safety, but because they minimize unnecessary suffering.

The argument for preparedness is not an appeal to a universal moral doctrine but to a minimal threshold of rationality that any functioning society already accepts in areas such as sanitation, electricity, fire safety, and public infrastructure. Cultures may differ in their philosophies of freedom or privacy, but no culture disputes the value of clean water, reliable medicine, or safe roads. Preparedness belongs to this same category: it is not an ethical imposition but a refusal to normalize preventable harm. The book does not claim that all societies must share identical moral principles; it claims only that when a civilization possesses the tools to prevent mass suffering at negligible cost, failing to use them is not cultural diversity—it is negligence. The duty to be ready is not a metaphysical commandment but the simplest form of collective sanity.

Even social insects—creatures with no philosophy, no politics, and no moral theories—maintain strict systems of sanitation and preventive readiness. Bees isolate infected individuals, remove contaminated material from the hive, and reorganize labor to contain outbreaks. Ants quarantine sick members, disinfect their pathways, and alter collective behavior to protect the colony. These species do not debate privacy, autonomy, or cultural preferences; they simply enact the biological logic of survival. When even a beehive recognizes the necessity of preparedness, the idea that human societies must first reconcile cultural differences before adopting preventive systems becomes absurd. Preparedness is not a moral imposition but a fundamental feature of any cooperative organism that intends to survive.

This moral dimension cannot be overstated. Every unprepared response is paid for in lives that could have been saved. The price of bureaucratic delay is measured not in spreadsheets but in grief. When technology exists to prevent predictable harm and we fail to deploy it, that failure is not neutral—it is ethical negligence. To build early warning systems, mobile care networks, robust supply chains, and secure health-data platforms is therefore not just a technical challenge but a moral commitment.

Preparedness is often dismissed as expensive, but so is regret. The economic and human cost of reactive crisis management dwarfs the investment required for anticipatory systems. The idea that readiness is extravagant belongs to the same era that treated pandemics as acts of fate rather than of governance. Civilization advanced the moment we stopped accepting famine, plague, and disaster as inevitable. That progress did not come from virtue alone, but from engineering: clean water, electricity, transportation, communication. Each was once a technological dream; now each is a moral expectation.

The next stage of civilization's moral evolution lies in our capacity to foresee and prevent systemic breakdown. The tools exist: artificial intelligence to model outbreaks, drones to deliver medicine, modular housing for rapid deployment, encrypted health-data networks for real-time coordination. What remains is the will to treat them not as gadgets or projects, but as public obligations—extensions of the social contract.

The book does not propose "permanent readiness" in the operational sense—no society can remain on high alert indefinitely, and no population can sustain motivation in the absence of visible threats. What it proposes is architectural readiness: systems that embed resilience by design, requiring no continuous psychological vigilance or political mobilization. A modular settlement pattern does not need to be motivated to disperse risk; an autonomous supply network does not need reminders to function; a unified medical database does not degrade because citizens stop thinking about pandemics. Like good sanitation, clean water systems, or fire codes, these structures operate quietly in the background, indifferent to the emotional state of society. Preparedness should not depend on perpetual tension but on infrastructure that remains ready precisely because its readiness is structural, not motivational.

Preparedness, in this light, is not a luxury of rich nations or an indulgence of technocrats. It is the minimum standard of care a society owes its people. To be technologically unprepared is to be ethically unprepared. And to build for resilience is to affirm, in the most practical sense possible, that civilization is worth the effort of continuation.

CHAPTER 1. PREPARING FOR A FUTURE PANDEMIC

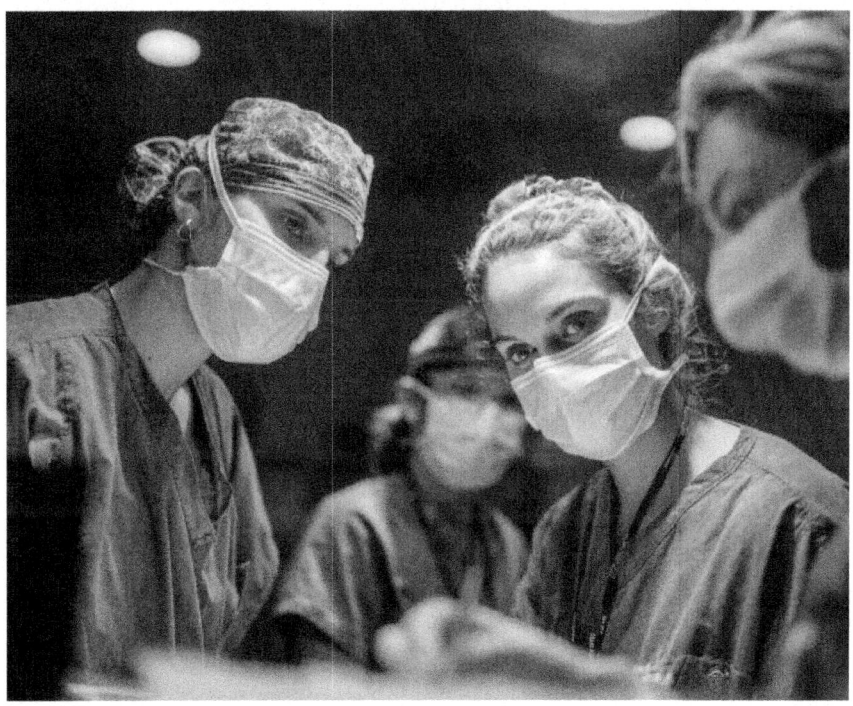

When the world was swept into the maelstrom of the coronavirus pandemic, I—like millions of others—watched the unfolding spectacle with a growing mix of horror, disappointment, and disbelief. It was as if humanity had collectively stumbled into a grotesque tragicomedy, a "theater of the absurd" played out on a global stage. There were moments when I thought to myself, half in jest, half in despair: *Perhaps I should write a book titled "CORONAPOCALYPSE: An Epidemic of*

Collective Idiocy." Because really, what could better capture the chaos of misinformation, the cacophony of panic, and the spectacle of good intentions drowned beneath waves of political grandstanding and mass hysteria?

But then a more sober thought followed: *Why add one more voice to the already deafening chorus of recriminations and post-mortems?* Every possible angle had been debated to exhaustion, every camp entrenched in its dogma as though defending the last fortress of reason. On one side, cries for personal freedom; on the other, calls for public safety. One faction insisted the virus was a lab-engineered menace, while another swore it leapt to humans from bats in a market. Some hailed vaccines as the triumph of science; others saw them as overpromised miracles that failed to meet expectations. Mask advocates fought with skeptics, quarantine supporters clashed with those who deemed lockdowns worse than the disease itself—and every camp viewed the others as heretical.

In the end, we didn't have public debate—we had ideological trench warfare. People no longer exchanged ideas; they exchanged accusations. Every discussion devolved into a shouting match between tribes convinced of their moral and intellectual superiority. Facts became secondary to identity, and science—once the great arbiter—was reduced to a prop in a political puppet show.

This, I realized, was the true contagion of our age: polarization. The virus infected our bodies, but dogma infected our minds. And so, instead of joining the fray, I decided to take a step back and wait for the dust to settle. What if, rather than arguing over who was right or wrong, we looked ahead? What if we used this global disaster as a mirror, reflecting everything broken in our systems, our institutions, and our collective psychology—and then tried to fix it before the next catastrophe arrives?

Because make no mistake: another catastrophe *will* come. Whether it's another virus, a climate disaster, a cyberwar, or even an extraterrestrial "first contact," we are just as unprepared for any of them as we were for COVID-19— which is to say, not at all.

The Collapse of Communication

One of the most catastrophic failures during the pandemic wasn't viral—it was informational. The world did not just suffer from a biological outbreak; it suffered from an outbreak of confusion. Critical data was delayed, distorted, or hidden. Misinformation spread faster than the virus itself. Governments, agencies, and hospitals operated in silos, duplicating efforts or missing crucial signals. Decisions were made blind, without reliable real-time insight into what was happening.

To prevent this in the future, we need more than new hospitals or stockpiles—we need an integrated *information ecosystem.* A system that ensures data is accurate, up-to-date, and immune to political or bureaucratic tampering. And here, modern technology—specifically artificial intelligence—offers an opportunity unprecedented in human history.

Imagine a healthcare infrastructure where AI continuously collects, analyzes, and interprets medical data from every corner of the system in real time. Instead of relying on fragmented reports or delayed statistics, decision-makers would have access to a living, breathing map of the nation's health.

AI systems can filter noise from truth, identify early warning signs of outbreaks, and predict where the next hotspot will emerge before it happens. They can compare regional hospital loads, flag anomalies in test results, and even assess the spread of misinformation itself—because in pandemics, disinformation can kill as effectively as disease.

Of course, such a system would demand rigorous protection of data privacy. Encryption, anonymization, and strict legal frameworks must safeguard personal information. But the potential benefits vastly outweigh the risks. To put it bluntly: a data leak may harm individuals, but the absence of data coordination can doom millions.

The Collapse of Communication

One of the most devastating failures of the coronavirus era was not biological at all—it was informational. The world did not merely face a pandemic; it faced a breakdown of communication so deep that it magnified every weakness in our systems. Governments, hospitals, research centers, and public-health agencies acted as if they inhabited different worlds, exchanging fragments instead of knowledge, delays instead of insight, and contradictions instead of coordination.

This failure is not an abstract claim. Its evidence is woven into the historical record. In England, a national backlog emerged when a large portion of newly reported positive tests simply vanished from the system because the central database relied on an outdated spreadsheet format with a maximum row limit. Tens of thousands of results were truncated; contact tracing stalled; the virus quietly advanced while authorities were looking at a distorted picture of reality. A single software decision—one rooted in bureaucracy, not biology—translated directly into preventable human infections.

Canada offers another example. The Auditor General reported that even before COVID-19, the national infectious-disease surveillance framework lacked finalized standards. Data moved slowly between provinces, formats differed, and responsibilities overlapped. When the pandemic hit, these structural seams tore open: regions could not see one another's burdens, federal systems lagged behind, and critical situational awareness arrived late or not at all.

At the global level, the World Health Organization formally recognized a new phenomenon: "the infodemic." Its definition was stark—misinformation spreading faster and more aggressively than any pathogen. The WHO was forced to establish dedicated teams, workflows, and strategies to track rumors, counter false narratives, and stabilize public perception. It was an acknowledgment that communication itself had become a parallel battlefield.

And yet, the counterexamples—though rare—proved what is possible. The Canadian company BlueDot, along with the global HealthMap monitoring system, detected the unusual pneumonia cluster in Wuhan on December 30–31, 2019, days before major institutions issued public alerts. These early warnings came not from political channels, but from AI-driven surveillance that scanned flight itineraries, hospital chatter, and local media reports around the world. In other words: the technology already worked, but the systems around it did not.

All of this points to the same conclusion. For future pandemics, merely building more hospitals or stockpiling supplies will not save us. What must be rebuilt is the informational foundation of public health. We need an integrated, real-time, cross-jurisdictional data ecosystem—one that no bureaucratic bottleneck and no political agenda can distort.

The elements of such an ecosystem already exist. Modern electronic health record systems can report data automatically using standardized formats such as HL7 FHIR, which were specifically created to allow different institutions to speak the same digital language. Public-health agencies already possess the technical guidelines for automated case reporting, validation, deduplication, and live dashboards. Artificial intelligence can serve as the analytical engine that transforms raw data into actionable insight: identifying anomalies, forecasting regional surges, detecting early signals of new outbreaks, and even monitoring the spread of misinformation by mapping how rumors propagate compared to case curves.

This is not technological fantasy. It is practical engineering.

Privacy concerns are often raised in response to proposals of this scale, and they deserve serious attention. But modern privacy engineering—anonymization, encryption, differential privacy, decentralized computation—allows us to protect individuals while still enabling society to defend itself. Even the Apple–Google exposure-notification framework demonstrated that it is possible to design a nationwide system where data stays on the user's device, cryptographically shielded, and still contributes to collective safety.

In crisis management, the true danger lies not in carefully engineered data sharing, but in its absence. A data leak may harm individuals; a data vacuum can harm entire nations.

Critics argue that such integrated systems could be abused by governments or misinterpreted by algorithms. The answer is not to avoid building them, but to build them with safeguards: transparent audit trails, independent oversight bodies, public documentation of algorithms, and clear limits on how data may be used. Bias and error are not reasons to abandon tools—they are reasons to measure, control, and correct them.

The cost argument also collapses upon inspection. The world has already paid the price for information failure—in missed contacts, misallocated resources, and shattered trust. The economic, social, and medical costs of flying blind exceeded, by magnitudes, the modest investment required to construct modern data infrastructure.

What is needed now is the will to treat communication as infrastructure.

Mandatory real-time reporting standards must be encoded in national law, not left to voluntary cooperation. Data pipelines must be automated, not stitched together during emergencies. Transparency must be non-negotiable: methodology changes, backfills, and errors should trigger public disclosures as reliably as alarms in an operating room. Above all, communication protocols must be rehearsed with the same seriousness as hospital triage or emergency logistics. When a data feed fails, when misinformation spikes, when public confidence wavers—there must be a playbook, not improvisation.

The lesson of COVID-19 is clear. A virus will challenge biology, but only we can choose whether confusion becomes its ally. Future preparedness begins not with fear, but with clarity. And clarity begins with a system where information flows as reliably as oxygen in a hospital: continuously, transparently, and protected by design.

The Case for a Unified Healthcare System

During the pandemic, hospitals were like islands—each struggling alone, blind to what the others were facing. A unified digital infrastructure, accessible across the entire healthcare network, would have changed everything.

Every patient's history, diagnosis, prescriptions, lab results, and physician notes could exist in a secure, cloud-based database—instantly available to authorized healthcare professionals. The duplication of tests, the loss of critical information, and the fatal delays in treatment could all be avoided.

Resource distribution would also be transformed. Ventilators, medications, and staff could be redirected based on real-time need, not guesswork. Predictive models could show where demand would surge days in advance, allowing preemptive action rather than reactive panic.

In essence, a unified system would act as the nervous system of national healthcare—fast, intelligent, and adaptive. It would save not only money but lives.

The United States provides some of the clearest proof that fragmentation in healthcare is not an inconvenience, but a structural danger. During COVID-19, the country's 6,000 hospitals operated on hundreds of incompatible electronic record systems. The Office of the Inspector General reported that many facilities could not share basic patient information—even between hospitals of the same chain—because their software systems lacked interoperability.

Critical data such as medications, allergies, ventilator settings, or prior test results often had to be reconstructed manually from patients or family members, or repeated entirely, wasting time and resources during the most critical phase of care.

In New York City, where hospitals were overwhelmed in March–April 2020, physicians resign themselves to repeating PCR tests and CT scans for transferred patients because the sending facility's records either could not be imported or arrived in unusable formats. A Columbia University analysis found that incomplete transfers of health records contributed directly to delays in triage, misallocation of limited ICU beds, and unnecessary exposure for staff who had to re-evaluate patients from scratch.

Ventilator distribution during the first wave exposed the same structural blindness. In early 2020, the federal government and the states had no unified real-time dashboard tracking ventilator availability; shipments were made based on phone calls, anecdotal reports, and political pressure. In some regions, unused ventilators sat in storage while other hospitals were improvising split-ventilation for two patients at once. A later review by the National Academies concluded that this chaos was the result of "absence of interoperable, real-time medical resource tracking"—exactly the gap a unified system would have prevented.

Even basic COVID case reporting suffered from this fragmentation. The CDC initially relied on fax machines, manual spreadsheets, and voluntary reporting by private laboratories. Some state health departments uploaded data to incompatible portals; others transmitted summary statistics without patient-level detail. As a result, national situational awareness lagged behind reality, and federal authorities often issued guidance based on outdated or incomplete information.

Underneath all of this lies the central problem: the United States does not have a national health information backbone. Instead, data lives in thousands of isolated silos—Epic here, Cerner there, proprietary systems everywhere—none of them mandated to interconnect. Hospitals were forced to fight with one hand tied, not because they lacked skill or courage, but because they lacked a common language.

The policy implications are clear. A unified system in the U.S. would require mandatory interoperability standards, a national cloud-based health record accessible through secure, audited channels, and federal authority to enforce uniform reporting formats. The legal framework already exists in fragments—the 21st Century Cures Act, federal interoperability rules, and HIPAA's provisions for data exchange—but none of them compel the creation of a single, coherent infrastructure. They merely encourage it, and "encouragement" predictably failed in an emergency.

Critics in the U.S. raise the familiar concerns: privacy, centralization, and "federal overreach." But these critiques ignore the reality exposed by the pandemic. Fragmentation did not protect privacy; instead, it forced clinicians to request sensitive information repeatedly, through insecure channels, during moments of crisis. Fragmentation did not prevent government misuse; it merely guaranteed government confusion. And fragmentation did not preserve state autonomy; it deprived states of the real-time intelligence needed to act effectively.

The architecture proposed in this book does not centralize power—it dissolves it. A unified medical database and national AI infrastructure are often imagined as instruments of control, but their function here is the opposite: to distribute decision-making across the smallest operational units and eliminate the bottlenecks that make centralized authority dangerous in the first place. Cluster-based settlement, autonomous logistics, and modular healthcare create a system with no single point of failure and no single point of domination. Power is not gathered at the top; it is fragmented by design. A government cannot control a society through systems that are decentralized, self-sufficient, and locally operable even when national institutions falter. The safeguards are not merely legal—they are architectural. By reducing dependency on central nodes, the system removes the very mechanisms through which abuse traditionally occurs.

A unified system does not require nationalizing hospitals

or erasing state authority. It requires only one thing: that the flow of life-saving information cannot depend on geography, software vendors, or institutional boundaries. The United States possesses some of the world's best clinicians, laboratories, and medical researchers. What it lacks—and what the pandemic proved it must build—is the shared digital nervous system that allows them to act as one organism instead of countless disjointed parts.

The reality of fragmented care during the pandemic is well documented. In Canada, federal auditors found that the healthcare system lacked a national framework for interoperable data; provinces used incompatible formats, and hospitals relied on separate, often outdated electronic record systems. As a result, clinicians frequently did not have access to a patient's full history, even within the same city. In the United States, the Office of the Inspector General reported that many hospitals could not transfer patient information during emergency surges because their electronic health record systems were not interlinked. These findings confirm that the "islands" you describe were not metaphorical—they were literal structural barriers embedded into the system.

The duplication of tests is also not hypothetical. Studies published after the first COVID-19 wave showed that patients transferred between facilities were routinely re-tested because prior results were not available or trusted. In some regions, as much as one quarter of PCR tests performed in hospitals were duplicates created solely because information did not travel with the patient. Delays in treatment followed the same pattern: missing medication lists caused avoidable drug interactions; unavailable imaging required repeating scans; ICU staff were often unaware of pre-existing conditions that would have changed clinical decisions.

A unified digital health system directly resolves these failures. Countries that already have centralized or near-centralized systems provide compelling empirical proof. Estonia's national health record, for example, allows physicians across the country to access imaging, prescriptions, and lab data within seconds; the system continued functioning even during heavy pandemic strain.

Denmark used its unified infrastructure to track ICU capacity nationally and move resources between regions before bottlenecks formed. In South Korea, real-time access to patient histories and contact-tracing data helped hospitals triage more effectively and reduced unnecessary admissions. The lesson is consistent across all these cases: **unified infrastructure increases accuracy, speed, and survival**.

Policy changes required to achieve this are straightforward, but must be uncompromising. A national mandate for interoperability should make a specific digital standard—such as HL7 FHIR—the legally required format for all medical systems. Hospitals should be funded to migrate legacy software into cloud-based architectures with secure, audited access controls. Every laboratory, clinic, pharmacy, and hospital must report structured data into a unified national platform, with penalties for non-compliance similar to those used for financial reporting. Resource-tracking modules—ventilators, medications, surgical capacity, staff availability—must be connected to the same platform so that resource distribution becomes an automated function of need, not telephone calls and improvisation.

The strongest critique against such a system is fear of surveillance and centralized vulnerability. But this argument collapses when examined carefully. First, medical systems already hold sensitive data; fragmentation does not reduce risk—it multiplies it. A unified system can use advanced encryption, fine-grained access logs, and zero-trust architecture, making unauthorized access traceable and punishable. Second, critics argue that concentration of data increases the impact of breaches, yet modern cloud systems run redundant, segmented databases where personal identifiers and clinical data can be split across independent layers. This makes breaches far less damaging than today's poorly protected, siloed hospital servers. Finally, some fear that governments may misuse the system. This is prevented by a legal framework that limits the purpose of data strictly to healthcare delivery and emergency planning, overseen by independent ethics boards with veto power over scope changes.

Resource-management critics may claim that predictive models cannot be trusted. Yet during the pandemic, predictive hospital-capacity models consistently outperformed manual estimates, and systems in Denmark and the Netherlands showed that early resource redistribution prevented collapses in local ICUs. The alternative is proven failure: guesswork, shortages, and last-minute appeals.

Opponents also argue that healthcare is too decentralized, administratively or constitutionally, for such a system to work. But unified digital infrastructure does not erase regional authority—it simply ensures that regions operate with shared information. A decentralized healthcare landscape is not incompatible with centralized knowledge; in fact, it depends on it for coordination.

The core truth remains: a unified healthcare system is not a luxury but a duty. It is the digital equivalent of clean water or electricity in a hospital—an invisible backbone without which modern medicine cannot function. The pandemic exposed what happens when that backbone is missing. Future preparedness demands that it finally be built.

Artificial Intelligence as the New Medic

Artificial intelligence, when properly integrated, could revolutionize not only data analysis but the practice of medicine itself. AI-driven diagnostics are already proving capable of detecting certain diseases faster and more accurately than human doctors. Given enough data, algorithms can identify subtle patterns that even experienced physicians might miss.

But AI's real potential lies in *democratization of care*. Through telemedicine platforms powered by intelligent systems, doctors can remotely consult patients anywhere on Earth, even in the most isolated regions. AI can help interpret symptoms, recommend preliminary tests, and suggest treatment options based on the patient's complete medical history.

In a world where hospitals themselves can become centers of contagion—as we saw during COVID-19—

telemedicine is not merely convenient; it is essential. AI-based monitoring tools can collect patient data from wearable sensors or smartphone applications, allowing continuous supervision without physical presence.

Imagine your phone acting as a pocket-sized diagnostic device—measuring blood pressure, oxygen levels, heart rhythm, and stress indicators. These metrics are analyzed instantly, and if an anomaly appears, both you and your doctor are alerted. With AI interpreting billions of such data points, diseases could be detected at their earliest stages, long before symptoms manifest.

Evidence already demonstrates that AI-driven diagnostics can outperform human clinicians in specific domains. The FDA has authorized autonomous AI systems capable of detecting diabetic retinopathy without a physician present, and large multicenter trials have shown that deep-learning models can identify lung cancer on CT scans earlier than radiologists with decades of experience. In dermatology, AI classifiers have reached accuracy levels comparable to expert dermatologists in detecting melanoma. These results confirm that the "subtle patterns" you describe are not theoretical: algorithms already identify micro-signatures invisible to the human eye.

Telemedicine, too, showed its value under pressure. During the early pandemic waves, U.S. medical consultations conducted via telehealth rose from under one percent to more than forty percent of all primary-care visits. In rural states—Montana, Wyoming, and parts of the Midwest—telemedicine became the only way many patients received ongoing care when hospitals were overwhelmed. Veterans Affairs, which operates one of the largest telemedicine networks in the country, reported that remote monitoring of chronic conditions prevented thousands of hospitalizations during COVID-19. These observations confirm that democratization of care is not an aspiration; it is something we have already witnessed when necessity forced adoption.

The vision of AI-enhanced remote diagnostics is equally grounded in existing technology. Wearable devices today routinely collect heart rate variability, arrhythmia episodes, blood oxygen saturation, sleep patterns, and mobility signatures. During the pandemic, researchers demonstrated that changes in wearable data—particularly heart-rate deviations and reduced activity—could predict COVID-19 infection days before symptoms appeared. Smartphone-based pulse oximetry and photoplethysmography systems are under clinical evaluation, and early results indicate that consumer devices can reliably measure oxygen saturation, detect atrial fibrillation, and identify stress-induced physiological shifts. The infrastructure for "pocket-sized diagnostics" therefore already exists; what is missing is standardized integration into healthcare workflows.

Policy changes must ensure clarity, responsibility, and safety. National regulators should establish certification pathways for AI diagnostic tools comparable to medical devices: transparent performance metrics, mandatory bias testing, post-market surveillance, and regular audits. Telemedicine reimbursement must be permanently codified, not treated as a temporary emergency measure; otherwise, the gains achieved during COVID-19 will evaporate. Legal frameworks must allow cross-state or cross-provincial licensing for remote consultations, so care is not restricted by geography. Healthcare providers must be funded to integrate continuous monitoring platforms, with patient consent and secure data-handling rules, into standard practice.

Critics often argue that AI will overstep its role, replace doctors, or make dangerous mistakes. Yet the strongest evidence contradicts this narrative. Autonomous AI systems currently approved in medicine are required to operate within narrow clinical bands with clear thresholds, error detection, and automatic referrals to human professionals when uncertainty is high. In most domains, AI serves as a second set of eyes—reducing oversight failures rather than increasing them. Another critique concerns bias: algorithms may perform poorly on underrepresented populations. This is addressed not by rejecting AI but by mandating diverse training datasets, publishing demographic performance reports, and requiring corrective updates when disparities appear. Regulatory oversight can enforce this in the same way safety recalls govern pharmaceuticals.

A philosophical critique claims that telemedicine reduces the human connection between doctor and patient. Yet, during the pandemic, remote consultations often preserved continuity of care when physical visits were impossible. Studies from large hospital systems showed that patient satisfaction with telemedicine equaled or exceeded traditional visits, particularly for chronic diseases, mental health, and primary-care management. Rather than weakening human care, AI-supported telemedicine can free physicians from administrative overload, giving them more time for the conversations, empathy, and judgment that no machine can replace.

Finally, privacy concerns are inevitable. But fragmentation does not protect privacy; it merely multiplies insecure storage points. Continuous monitoring systems can be built around encryption, anonymized identifiers, and on-device preprocessing, where only relevant alerts—not raw biometric streams—are transmitted. Zero-knowledge architectures already exist for financial and cryptographic systems; applying them to health data is a technical extension, not a conceptual leap.

Taken together, these facts reveal that AI is not a futuristic intrusion into medicine—it is the next logical advance after stethoscopes, imaging, and laboratory diagnostics. When integrated responsibly, it expands the reach of physicians, strengthens early detection, and shields both patients and healthcare workers from unnecessary exposure. The pandemic showed the fragility of physical proximity; the future will be shaped by intelligent systems that preserve care even when distance is a necessity.

There is ample evidence that professional resistance to AI adoption in medicine is not driven by malice, but by entrenched incentives. Clinical reimbursement systems in the United States reward in-person visits, procedures, and specialty interventions far more than remote monitoring or automated screening. This creates a structural economic barrier: every diagnostic test performed by an algorithm, every preliminary triage handled remotely, and every chronic condition managed through continuous AI-supported monitoring represents revenue that shifts away from traditional billing models. When systems reward volume rather than outcomes, it is rational—not ethical—

for institutions and practitioners to guard the status quo.

Empirical studies show this pattern clearly. Before the pandemic, telemedicine adoption in the U.S. remained below one percent despite decades of technological capability. The barrier was not technical feasibility but reimbursement: insurers simply did not pay for virtual visits on equal terms. Only when COVID-19 emergency measures forced payment parity did telemedicine usage explode to over forty percent of primary-care encounters. Once emergency waivers expired, many providers lobbied to limit or roll back telehealth equivalence. The same dynamic appears with AI diagnostics: autonomous diabetic retinopathy systems approved in the United States have been adopted slowly because they shift part of the diagnostic value chain away from specialists.

Patient resistance comes from a different mechanism. Most patients cannot evaluate medical quality directly; they rely on symbolic proxies—white coats, personal impressions, or institutional branding. Numerous studies reveal that patients routinely overestimate the accuracy of human diagnosis and underestimate the reliability of algorithmic interpretation. This cognitive bias persists even in controlled experiments where participants are shown explicit accuracy statistics demonstrating that AI performs better. The resistance is therefore psychological, not empirical: a preference for the familiar over the demonstrably superior.

To address professional resistance, policy must realign incentives in favor of outcomes, not procedures. Payment systems should reward accurate diagnosis, early detection, and reduction of hospitalizations—areas where AI excels. If financial structures shift toward value-based reimbursement, practitioners will see AI not as a threat but as a tool to meet performance targets. Mandatory reporting of diagnostic accuracy could also drive adoption: when human performance is publicly measured against algorithmic alternatives, the pressure to use better tools becomes ethical, not optional.

Patient resistance requires a different approach. Systems that integrate AI must be transparent about how decisions are made, offer clear explanations, and demonstrate reliability through consistent, reproducible outcomes.

Public communication campaigns can play the same role they once did for vaccines and sanitation: normalizing the idea that algorithmic second opinions are not replacements for physicians but safeguards against the limitations of human perception.

Critics may argue that this line of reasoning paints physicians as self-interested. But the more accurate framing is that the existing system forces them to behave as rational actors within flawed incentive structures. Resistance is not a moral failure; it is a predictable outcome of a system that financially rewards the old model. The better critique is that societies must build systems where economic and clinical incentives point in the same direction.

Another common objection asserts that AI lacks empathy, context, or holistic judgment. Yet evidence shows that most diagnostic failures are not failures of empathy but failures of pattern recognition, incomplete information, or cognitive overload—areas where AI has measurable advantages. Empathy remains vital, but it is not diminished by the presence of an algorithm that catches what the clinician may miss.

A final critique argues that AI dehumanizes medicine. The reality is the opposite. In systems where AI handles monitoring, preliminary analysis, and routine screening, physicians spend less time on clerical tasks and more time speaking with patients. In this sense, AI acts as a force that restores the human element medicine has gradually lost.

When viewed through evidence and incentives rather than sentiment, it becomes clear why resistance emerges and why it must be addressed not through confrontation but through structural reform. A healthcare system aligned with truth and outcomes will naturally embrace the tools that elevate both.

Drones: The Skyborne Lifeline

Another lesson from the pandemic: logistics can be as deadly as the disease. Delays in delivering medication, tests, and supplies cost lives. Entire regions were effectively cut off due to quarantines or infrastructure breakdowns. Here again, technology offers a solution that is both simple and revolutionary—*drones*.

Autonomous aerial delivery can provide safe, contactless transportation of medicines, vaccines, and biological samples. Drones can reach mountain villages, remote islands, or quarantined zones without risking human contact. They can deliver insulin to a diabetic patient hundreds of miles away or carry swab samples from a rural clinic to a city lab in minutes instead of hours.

Beyond efficiency, drones represent resilience. They can operate when roads are blocked, airports closed, or cities locked down. In the next crisis, drone logistics may prove as critical as ventilators or vaccines.

Real-world experience already proves the reliability of drone logistics. Rwanda and Ghana became the first countries to integrate medical drones into their national healthcare systems years before the pandemic, using autonomous aircraft to deliver blood, vaccines, and antivenom across difficult terrain. During COVID-19, these same systems continued operating even when ground transport collapsed, making thousands of deliveries that would otherwise have been impossible. In the United States, the FAA granted emergency waivers to allow medical drone shipments in North Carolina, where hospital networks used autonomous flights to transport PPE, COVID test kits, and laboratory samples between campuses—cutting delivery times by up to 80 percent. In Ireland, drones delivered medications to elderly patients in coastal areas when ferry transport shut down. These examples confirm that drones do not merely promise resilience—they have already demonstrated it.

The biological-sample advantage is especially compelling. For many pathogens, the value of test results decays by the hour. During the early pandemic, rural clinics in dozens of countries experienced turnaround times of two to five days due to distance and courier shortages. Drone transport compresses that window dramatically and improves diagnostic accuracy simply by preserving sample viability. The same applies to emergency medications: epinephrine, insulin, and antiretrovirals have already been delivered by drones under controlled, temperature-stabilized conditions in field programs.

Policy changes must make this capacity permanent rather than experimental. Aviation authorities need clear regulatory corridors for medical drone operations: designated low-altitude routes, pre-authorized emergency flight zones, and simplified approval mechanisms during public-health crises. National healthcare systems should contract with drone operators the way they contract with ambulance providers—creating a standing, ready-to-deploy fleet rather than improvising during crises. Medical supply chains must be redesigned so that distribution centers automatically trigger drone dispatch when certain thresholds are reached, instead of depending on human scheduling.

Critics often claim that drones are unreliable during bad weather or too limited in payload. Yet the most advanced medical drones already operate in rain, wind, and nighttime conditions, and their payload capacity now regularly exceeds 2–5 kilograms—sufficient for most critical medications, vaccines, blood units, and laboratory samples. For heavier loads, hybrid fixed-wing models and electric-VTOL aircraft are being deployed in pilot programs. Logistics does not need drones to replace trucks or airplanes; it needs them to complement those systems where fragility is highest: the last mile, blocked corridors, quarantine zones, and time-critical deliveries.

Another critique argues that drones raise privacy concerns. But medical drones need not carry cameras at all; many already use radar, GPS, LiDAR, or inertial navigation without any visual recording. Unlike surveillance drones, delivery drones can be engineered to collect zero imagery and to store no personal information beyond a destination coordinate. In many ways, they reduce privacy risks by eliminating the need for human couriers who handle sensitive materials.

Finally, some question economic feasibility. Yet global analyses consistently show that drone transport becomes cost-efficient precisely in the scenarios where traditional logistics fails: remote regions, emergency deliveries, dispersed populations, or disaster zones. A single avoided helicopter flight for blood transport pays for entire fleets of drones.

In the next crisis, the difference between a two-hour delay and a fifteen-minute flight may decide survival. Drone logistics will not replace hospitals or ambulances—but they will ensure that medicine itself can still move when the world cannot.

Redesigning Society: Urban Dispersal and Resilience

But technology alone is not enough. We must also rethink the very structure of our civilization. The pandemic revealed how vulnerable modern urban life is—how quickly dense populations can become petri dishes for contagion. Cities, once symbols of progress, turned into pressure cookers of infection.

The solution is not isolation, but *dispersion*: modular, decentralized urban design. Imagine small, self-sufficient residential clusters—connected by existing road networks, each equipped with local power generation, medical pods, and digital infrastructure. In such a model, society remains connected yet physically diffused, minimizing the speed of viral transmission without sacrificing economic or social cohesion.

This concept of "urban modularity" isn't just about public health. It could also mitigate traffic congestion, reduce pollution, and improve mental well-being. Humanity, after all, was never meant to live stacked like sardines in glass towers.

The fragility of hyper-dense cities has been quantified repeatedly. During the first waves of COVID-19, New York, London, Milan, and São Paulo displayed the same pattern: transmission accelerated fastest in districts with high residential density, overcrowded transit, and limited living space. In New York City, ZIP codes with the greatest population density experienced hospitalization rates two to three times higher than less dense boroughs, even after adjusting for socioeconomic factors. Epidemiologists documented a simple structural truth: the more tightly people live, the more the virus exploits the geometry of their lives.

Decentralization already has precedents. After the 2011

earthquake and tsunami, Japan accelerated experiments with "compact smart towns"—small, modular communities connected digitally to larger hubs, designed to withstand disasters without collapsing into chaos. In the Netherlands, several municipalities have trialed "distributed living clusters," where housing, renewable power, workspace, and medical facilities are arranged in walkable micro-neighborhoods. These communities demonstrated greater resilience during the pandemic because residents could access essential services within their immediate area, reducing reliance on crowded transport and centralized urban cores.

The infrastructure for modular living does not require constructing new cities; it requires repurposing what already exists. The vast strips of unused roadside land, underdeveloped peri-urban belts, and declining industrial zones are natural candidates for modular housing units—lightweight, quickly deployable, energy-efficient, and easily connected to digital networks. Modern prefabricated homes, autonomous micro-clinics, solar arrays, and water-recycling systems make these clusters not theoretical but technologically practical.

Policy reforms must focus on zoning, incentives, and infrastructure integration. Governments should create "modular development corridors" along existing highways, where micro-communities can be installed without triggering years-long planning battles. Building codes need new categories for high-efficiency modular dwellings, allowing faster approvals and standardized safety requirements. Grid operators should provide microgrid interconnection frameworks enabling communities to run semi-independently during crises. And healthcare systems must deploy decentralized telemedicine pods, staffed physically only when needed but maintained as part of the national digital health backbone.

Critics argue that dispersion threatens economic density and cultural vibrancy. Yet the pandemic exposed the opposite: productivity in many industries remained stable or even increased as millions shifted to remote or hybrid work. What collapsed were not economic relationships, but outdated assumptions about where people must physically gather. Cultural life, likewise, adapts to digital platforms without disappearing; dispersion does not eliminate community—it changes its geometry.

Another critique warns of urban sprawl and environmental damage. But modular dispersal is not sprawl; it is structured decentralization. It replaces endless low-density expansion with intentionally designed clusters that use renewable energy, local food production, and digital services to reduce ecological footprint. A well-planned modular system requires less land per capita than traditional suburban development and dramatically less energy than skyscraper-based city centers.

A final objection insists that humans prefer dense, vibrant cities. Historical evidence suggests otherwise. Across millennia, most human settlements consisted of small clusters—villages, communes, hamlets, or districts within larger towns. Only in the last century did vertical megacity living become widespread, driven by industrial economics rather than biological or psychological well-being. Surveys during the pandemic showed rising interest in greener, quieter, more spacious living environments. Dispersion does not fight human nature; it acknowledges it.

Redesigning society through modular dispersal is not an abandonment of civilization but an evolution of it. Technology gives us powerful tools; urban modularity gives us a resilient structure in which those tools can operate. Together, they form a blueprint for a society that remains connected, prosperous, and humane—even in the face of the next global disruption.

Urban dispersal is not merely a pandemic-era precaution; it is a solution to a vast constellation of systemic problems that predate COVID-19 and will outlast it. Modern megacities suffer from chronic ailments that no amount of traditional urban planning has managed to cure. Traffic congestion alone consumes billions of hours of human life every year. Air pollution in dense metropolitan areas shortens life expectancy more reliably than many infectious diseases. Housing shortages in global cities have driven home prices far beyond affordability, creating conditions where entire generations remain trapped in rental cycles with no prospect of stability. Mental-health data reveal another dimension: rates of anxiety, depression, and burnout are consistently higher in the densest urban centers, where sensory overload, constant crowds, and environmental stressors shape daily existence.

Decentralized living directly addresses these structural deficits. Smaller modular communities reduce traffic by shortening travel distances and distributing economic activity across a broader geographic field. With local energy systems—solar arrays, battery storage, and microgrids—clusters become less dependent on vulnerable centralized grids, which themselves are increasingly threatened by aging infrastructure and extreme weather. Local food production, including vertical micro-farms and community agriculture pods, strengthens food security at a time when global supply chains are repeatedly disrupted by geopolitical instability. Modular medical pods, integrated into a national digital backbone, improve access to care for rural and underserved populations even outside of crisis conditions.

The benefits reach deep into social and economic life.

Dispersal alleviates the urban housing crisis simply by expanding the geography of livable space without resorting to endless high-rise development. It provides young families, elders, and low-income workers options that do not force them into overcrowded apartments or multi-hour commutes. It also reduces inequality: when services and opportunities are spread across a wider network instead of concentrated in exclusive urban cores, access becomes more democratic, not less. Crime patterns shift as well. Numerous studies show that hyper-dense urban districts experience higher rates of violent crime, while smaller, community-scaled environments foster stronger social cohesion and lower crime rates through natural neighborhood oversight.

Environmental resilience is another pillar of the argument. Climate change has made cities increasingly vulnerable to floods, heatwaves, electrical grid failures, and infrastructure collapses. Modular clusters, powered by decentralized energy and built with resilient materials, are far easier to protect and restore after extreme events. In wildfire-prone regions, distributed settlements reduce the catastrophic impact of fire sweeping through single corridors of dense habitation. In flood zones, modular homes can be elevated, relocated, or replaced with a fraction of the cost required to retro-engineer entire urban districts.

From an economic perspective, dispersal increases national flexibility. The global shift toward remote and hybrid work has already demonstrated that productivity does not depend on daily physical congregation in commercial towers. If anything, decentralization reduces overhead costs, distributes consumption, and revitalizes regions previously excluded from economic development. Entire towns that had been declining for decades have begun to regrow when remote professionals relocate, bringing new economic life without the burden of building massive centralized infrastructure.

Critics fear that dispersal will dilute culture or weaken innovation clusters. But history shows that creativity flourishes in diversity, not in overcrowding. The most innovative regions are not necessarily the densest, but the ones with strong digital connectivity, high quality of life, and mobility between clusters of talent. In a modular society, ideas travel as easily as data; collaboration is a matter of connectivity, not geography.

The deeper truth is this: urban modularity is not a retreat from civilization but its modernization. It is a recognition that the 20th-century urban model—designed around factories, skyscrapers, and mass commuting—no longer fits the realities of the 21st century: digital economies, remote work, ecological constraints, and global volatility. Dispersal is not merely a health measure; it is an architectural correction, an ecological adjustment, and a social recalibration.

A society built on modular, decentralized principles becomes not only pandemic-resistant but cleaner, calmer, safer, more equitable, and more adaptable. It restores the human scale of living without sacrificing the power of a connected civilization.

The New World of Work

Another seismic shift sparked by the pandemic was the redefinition of work itself. The forced mass experiment in remote employment revealed a truth long ignored: much of the modern office was a ritual, not a necessity. The ability to work from anywhere shattered the old geography of labor.

However, to make remote work sustainable, nations need coherent legal frameworks that protect both employers and employees. Companies must provide the necessary digital tools and cybersecurity, while workers must have the right to balanced hours and data protection. Properly managed, remote work could enhance productivity, broaden access to global talent, and reduce carbon emissions from commuting.

It's not just a matter of convenience—it's a matter of resilience. A world where economies can continue functioning amid lockdowns or disasters is a world better prepared for whatever comes next.

The global experiment of 2020–2021 delivered a verdict that decades of theory never dared to state openly. Across the United States, Canada, the United Kingdom, and much of Europe, productivity did not collapse when office towers emptied; in many sectors, it reached heights not recorded in years. A major Stanford study found that remote employees outperformed their office-bound counterparts by measurable margins, largely because the noise, interruptions, and exhaustion of daily commuting vanished from their lives. Corporate data echoed the same pattern: work did not deteriorate—it sharpened. What the pandemic revealed was a truth obscured by habit. The modern office, with its open-plan distractions and ritualistic presence requirements, belonged to an industrial past rather than a digital present.

This transformation extended far beyond individual output. The geography of labor itself shifted. Companies suddenly discovered talent in places they had never looked: rural towns, remote regions, small communities far from traditional corporate centers. Workers who once lived outside the gravitational pull of major cities found themselves participating in national and even global labor markets. The dispersion of opportunity softened regional inequalities and breathed new life into areas previously dismissed as economically peripheral.

Yet the shift also exposed the regulatory vacuum underlying the old system. Labor laws built for physical workplaces proved unfit for a dispersed workforce. Clear working hours blurred into endless availability. Homes became offices without legal protections or compensation. Digital surveillance crept into daily life. Meanwhile, employers faced their own uncertainties: cybersecurity responsibilities, equipment obligations, and jurisdictional ambiguities when employees worked across state or national borders. The world of work had changed, but the rules governing it had not.

A coherent framework is essential. Modern labor policy must rest on several pillars: the right to disconnect, ensuring that remote work does not silently become perpetual work; guaranteed digital infrastructure and secure equipment provided or funded by employers; clear cross-jurisdictional standards that specify which laws apply to remote employees; and the replacement of presence-based evaluation with outcome-based metrics aligned with the realities of digital labor.

Some nations have already begun to adapt. France and Portugal recognize the right to disconnect as a legal protection. Germany has moved toward requiring employer-funded equipment for remote workers. Estonia has pioneered digital residency models that allow cross-border labor to operate within a stable legal envelope. These examples show that remote work can be regulated without eroding either flexibility or fairness.

Critics insist that distance undermines creativity, collaboration, or corporate culture. Yet experience from hybrid organizations demonstrates the opposite. When people gather by intention rather than compulsion, meetings become sharper, less wasteful, and more purposeful. Creativity thrives when communication is deliberate, not constant. The true obstacles to innovation—poor leadership, vague expectations, and misaligned processes—long predated remote work and merely surfaced when the crutches of physical proximity disappeared.

Concerns about isolation are legitimate, but not inherent

to decentralized work. Properly structured hybrid schedules, community coworking hubs, and regular team rituals restore social connection while preserving the advantages of flexibility. Remote work expands human choice; it does not abolish social life.

Economic anxieties about empty city centers also overlook the capacity of cities to reinvent themselves. Commercial districts can evolve into residential neighborhoods, cultural spaces, modular healthcare hubs, and green corridors. The long-term gains—lower emissions, shorter commutes, revitalized regional economies, and expanded workforce participation—far exceed the temporary dislocation of transition.

Remote work is not an emergency improvisation but a structural evolution. It strengthens resilience by ensuring that economic activity can continue when pandemics, natural disasters, or infrastructural crises strike. It broadens opportunity, improves well-being, and aligns daily life with the realities of a digital civilization. Societies that embrace this transformation will not merely endure the next global shock—they will outpace those still clinging to outdated geography.

Toward a Smarter Civilization

Preparing for the next pandemic—or any global crisis—requires more than vaccines and stockpiles. It demands a reinvention of our systems, guided by intelligence, technology, and pragmatism. It means shifting focus from reaction to prevention, from centralization to intelligent decentralization, from panic to preparedness.

If we can create integrated healthcare systems, powered by artificial intelligence, enhanced by drones, and supported by flexible social structures, humanity will not only survive the next crisis—it will evolve through it.

Because the real lesson of the coronavirus was never about a virus at all. It was about us—our arrogance, our complacency, and our failure to learn. The next pandemic will test not just our immune systems but our capacity for wisdom. And this time, ignorance will not be an excuse.

A truly intelligent civilization is one that refuses to repeat its mistakes. The coronavirus era exposed a pattern that has recurred throughout human history: societies respond passionately to disasters but rarely transform themselves afterward. Hurricanes lead to temporary vigilance, then complacency. Financial crises spark reforms, then slow decay into old habits. Pandemics ignite global fear, then are quietly forgotten the moment headlines shift. The only way to break this cycle is to redesign the very architecture of collective life, so that preparedness becomes a structural feature, not an emotional reaction.

Resilience begins long before a pathogen emerges. It begins in supply chains that can reroute themselves automatically when borders close, in digital infrastructures that remain functional when physical mobility collapses, and in governance models that replace bureaucratic inertia with real-time intelligence. The nations that weathered the pandemic most effectively were not those with the largest stockpiles but those with the most adaptable systems—countries where health data flowed quickly, where logistics could pivot overnight, and where public communication was coherent instead of chaotic.

Intelligent decentralization becomes the key to this adaptability. Instead of concentrating everything in fragile megastructures—mega-hospitals, mega-cities, mega-bureaucracies—a wiser civilization distributes its strength. It places diagnostic capacity in every home, telemedicine in every pocket, modular clinics along highways, and supply hubs capable of autonomous operation. It does not rely on heroics; it relies on architecture. When resilience is engineered into daily life, crises no longer require extraordinary improvisation. They simply activate the systems already in place.

Such a transformation extends beyond healthcare. Energy grids capable of operating as microgrids can isolate failures and prevent cascading blackouts. Education systems built around hybrid learning can continue uninterrupted during disasters. Judicial systems designed for digital operation can maintain continuity without forcing citizens into physical spaces. Even democracy itself becomes more resilient when secure digital voting infrastructures eliminate the bottleneck of physical presence.

The deeper implication is that humanity must finally abandon the superstition that the world can be managed by intuition alone. Contemporary civilization is too complex, too interconnected, and too fast-moving for governance by analog instincts. Intelligence—both artificial and institutional—must be embedded into every public system. This does not diminish human agency; it strengthens it. When algorithms handle what is mechanical, humans regain the freedom to focus on what requires judgment, compassion, and imagination.

Critics argue that such a transformation risks overreliance on technology. Yet the pandemic demonstrated the opposite: societies collapsed not because technology failed but because technology was absent where it was needed most. The fragility came from inefficiency, not from innovation. True resilience lies not in rejecting the modern world but in harnessing it fully, consciously, and ethically.

The test ahead is not merely biological. It is moral. A

civilization willing to learn will redesign its systems to protect life; a civilization clinging to outdated structures will repeat the tragedy. Humanity now stands at the threshold where wisdom becomes a survival strategy. The next crisis—whether viral, climatic, economic, or political—will measure our capacity to evolve. And evolution, unlike disaster, is always a choice.

CHAPTER 2. LESSONS IN RESILIENCE: BUILDING A SMARTER WORLD AFTER THE PANDEMIC

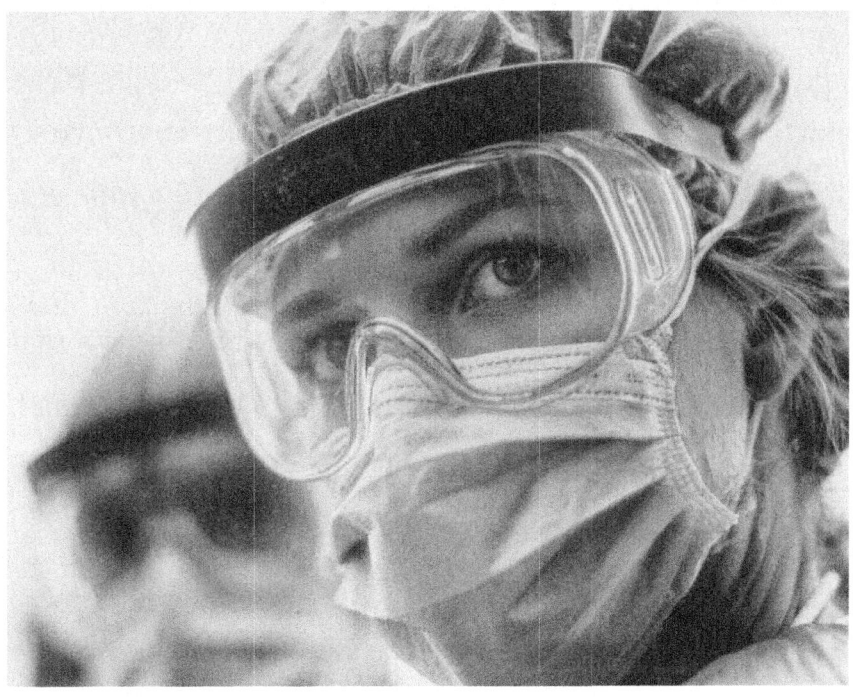

When the long shadow of the pandemic began to recede, one might have expected that humanity—having paid such a colossal price—would emerge wiser. Yet, almost as soon as the fear faded, the old habits returned. Offices reopened, cubicles were dusted off, and governments, along with many private employers, seemed desperate to herd people back into the same fluorescent-lit spaces they had once fled.

It was a curious sight, as though we had collectively learned nothing. The insistence on returning to pre-pandemic office routines brought with it a familiar catalogue of frustrations—commutes that devour hours, traffic that gnaws at sanity, and the slow erosion of work-life balance that remote work had, for a fleeting moment, made possible.

Remote work had shown us something extraordinary: that trust, autonomy, and technology could coexist. Productivity did not collapse when people stayed home— it often improved. Parents could see their children at lunchtime; employees could work from quiet corners instead of chaotic open offices; and countless tons of carbon emissions vanished from the atmosphere as rush hours dissolved into memory. For a brief, shining moment, the modern world glimpsed what a truly flexible society might look like.

But nostalgia for control runs deep. Managers longed for the illusion of oversight, for the ability to "see" work being done, as though presence equaled productivity. Bureaucracies, allergic to change, demanded the old rituals of attendance and paperwork. The result was a retreat from progress—a failure to capitalize on one of the most profound social experiments of the modern era.

Reverting to physical offices didn't just burden workers; it strained economies. Companies faced renewed costs for office leases, maintenance, and commuting subsidies—expenses that could have been redirected toward innovation, technology, or employee well-being. What could have been a turning point for the modernization of work became instead a relapse into inertia.

Reinventing Supply Chains for an Uncertain World

If the pandemic taught us anything, it was that our global supply chains—the hidden arteries of civilization—were fragile to the point of absurdity. A microscopic virus grounded airplanes, emptied supermarket shelves, and exposed just how dependent the modern world is on just-in-time production and a handful of manufacturing regions.

To survive future crises, we must reimagine supply chains

as *living systems*: flexible, transparent, and adaptive. That means diversification—no more placing all of humanity's eggs in a single industrial basket. Relying on one supplier or one region for critical goods like medicines, food, or medical equipment is a recipe for catastrophe.

A resilient system must combine global reach with local capacity. This can be achieved by developing multiple backup supply lines, encouraging regional production hubs, and maintaining strategic reserves of essentials. Redundancy, once considered wasteful, must now be recognized as the price of survival.

Technology will be the backbone of this transformation. Artificial intelligence can analyze supply and demand in real time, anticipate shortages, and propose corrective actions before crises spiral out of control. Blockchain technology, meanwhile, can bring transparency to every link in the chain, allowing goods to be tracked from producer to consumer. The result is not only efficiency but trust—an antidote to panic when things go wrong.

Governments, too, must play their part by maintaining national stockpiles of vital goods: food, medicine, fuel, protective equipment, and even raw materials. These reserves, intelligently managed and regularly rotated, can prevent the kind of shortages that turn crises into disasters.

And logistics—the unsung hero of every functioning society—must evolve. The future lies in automation: drone deliveries to isolated areas, AI-managed warehouses that restock themselves, and smart transportation networks that reroute dynamically when disruptions occur. These are not science fiction dreams but necessary adaptations for a century in which unpredictability will be the norm.

The collapse of global supply lines during the pandemic was not an anomaly but the predictable consequence of a system designed for maximum efficiency at the cost of all resilience. For decades, just-in-time manufacturing had been celebrated as a masterpiece of modern economics: inventories reduced to the bare minimum, factories synchronized across continents, and supply routes optimized to the second. Yet beneath this elegance lay a fatal vulnerability. A single disruption—be it a virus, a war, a shipping accident, or a climate disaster—was capable of bringing entire industries to a standstill. When a single container ship blocked the Suez Canal, billions were lost in less than a week. When one region shut its ports, medical masks and critical components disappeared worldwide.

This fragility revealed a deeper truth: a civilization that relies on uninterrupted global motion is a civilization that has forgotten the meaning of interruption. The future will not allow such forgetfulness. Climate instability, geopolitical tensions, cyberattacks, and resource scarcity guarantee that disruptions will no longer be rare events but recurring features of the century ahead. The supply chains that served the calm decades of globalization cannot survive the storms of the coming age.

Resilience begins with structural redesign. Distributed manufacturing must replace monocentric dependence. Emerging technologies—3D printing, precision robotics, modular micro-factories—enable production to be spread across multiple regions rather than concentrated in a single industrial corridor. Nations can manufacture critical components locally while still participating in global trade, creating a hybrid model where autonomy and interdependence reinforce rather than contradict each other.

Strategic reserves must evolve beyond static warehouses filled with dust-covered supplies. They should operate as dynamic ecosystems: rotating stock to prevent expiration, analyzing consumption patterns, forecasting seasonal vulnerabilities, and automatically replenishing critical materials long before shortages arise. Some countries have already begun to adopt this model, transforming their national reserves into living institutions capable of responding to real-time signals.

Transparency is equally essential. During the pandemic, confusion over where goods were produced, how much existed, and who controlled access created unnecessary chaos. A supply chain without visibility becomes fertile ground for rumors, price gouging, and political manipulation. Blockchain systems—properly implemented, without the noise of speculative hype— offer a simple solution: an immutable ledger that records every movement of critical goods, ensuring that no single actor can conceal, hoard, or misreport stock without detection.

Logistics will undergo a parallel transformation. Automated warehouses capable of twenty-four-hour operation reduce the bottlenecks that plagued traditional distribution centers. Electric autonomous trucks can move goods even when driver shortages or curfews halt conventional transport. Hybrid rail-road systems, predictive port management, and decentralized delivery hubs create a landscape where goods do not depend on fragile chokepoints. In remote areas or during lockdowns, fleets of drones can maintain lifelines when roads fail or human movement becomes dangerous.

Critics claim that redundancy is too expensive. Yet the true cost of fragility—the trillions lost during a single global crisis—dwarfs the price of strategic foresight. Robust systems appear costly only in times of stability; in times of crisis, they are priceless. The logic is simple: resilience is an investment, not an expense.

Others argue that decentralization threatens the efficiencies gained from global integration. But the aim is not to dismantle globalization—it is to anchor it in realism. A world that balances global reach with local capability becomes more stable, not less. Diversity strengthens ecosystems; it also strengthens economies.

The ultimate lesson is that supply chains must cease being invisible. They must be recognized as the vital organs of civilization, deserving of the same protection, intelligence, and redundancy that societies reserve for healthcare, energy, and national security. A future defined by uncertainty demands systems capable of bending without breaking. Only by embracing this truth can humanity ensure that the next disruption—whatever its form—does not unravel the fabric of modern life.

The Case for Mobile Medicine

Healthcare, too, must learn to move. The pandemic revealed the limits of static hospital systems built for routine, not emergency. When hospitals overflowed, patients were left untreated; when infections surged in one region, resources in another sat idle.

Enter the concept of *mobile healthcare capacity*—a network of modular, deployable hospitals and medical units capable of rapid response anywhere, anytime. These mobile hospitals could be transported and assembled within hours, fully equipped for diagnostics, treatment, and intensive care. In times of crisis, they would function as autonomous lifelines, bringing medicine to the front lines rather than forcing patients to travel to overburdened cities.

Strategic positioning of these mobile units would allow them to be deployed to emerging hotspots, natural disaster zones, or refugee camps. Complementary mobile laboratories could handle on-site testing, ensuring that diagnosis and containment happen faster than the spread of infection.

Such systems could be supported by telemedicine networks, allowing specialists to remotely consult and guide local teams. Doctors could treat dozens of patients across continents from a single console. Combined with AI diagnostics and real-time data analysis, mobile healthcare could become as dynamic as the crises it confronts.

This vision demands investment, of course—but far less than the economic damage of unpreparedness. Every mobile hospital deployed in time could prevent thousands of deaths and millions in economic losses. It is the kind of investment that pays for itself many times over, in both lives and resilience.

The concept of mobile medicine is not speculative; it has already proven itself whenever rigid systems falter. During the early months of COVID-19, countries that deployed flexible medical capacity fared significantly better at stabilizing surges. China's rapid construction and deployment of modular hospitals in Wuhan—assembled in days, not months—demonstrated how mobility can transform the trajectory of an outbreak. Italy, overwhelmed by simultaneous regional waves, relied on military field hospitals that restored critical care capacity where it was collapsing. Even the United States mobilized naval medical ships and converted stadiums into temporary wards, though the speed and efficiency of these efforts were constrained by bureaucratic friction and technological fragmentation. These experiences offered a clear message: when care becomes mobile, survival becomes possible.

Yet the potential of mobile medicine extends far beyond emergency tents or improvised wards. Modern modular hospital systems can be manufactured in standardized units—sterile modules for intensive care, surgical pods, imaging suites, and laboratory compartments—that lock together like engineered architecture. Equipped with negative-pressure rooms, autonomous power generation, and integrated oxygen and filtration systems, they can operate independently even in devastated or remote regions. Their deployment no longer requires weeks of construction or convoys of specialists; the modules themselves carry the infrastructure.

A mobile healthcare network transforms national capacity into something fluid rather than fixed. Instead of static hospitals that become overwhelmed while others remain underused, an entire country gains the ability to shift capacity like an intelligent organism responding to stress.

When wildfires, hurricanes, or floods destroy physical infrastructure, mobile hospitals can stand in its place. When mass migration or refugee crises erupt, they can provide stable care where none exists. When epidemics appear at borders or remote crossings, mobile laboratories can prevent local sparks from becoming national infernos.

The integration of telemedicine elevates these capabilities. A specialist in neurology, cardiology, oncology, or infectious disease can guide frontline teams from thousands of kilometers away. Remote robotic ultrasound, AI-assisted imaging interpretation, and wearable biometric streams allow complex diagnostics to occur even when physical specialists are absent. For nations with vast rural territories or limited specialist distribution, this fusion of mobility and telepresence collapses the tyranny of distance.

These systems also redefine preparedness. Instead of stockpiling only masks and ventilators, nations can stockpile entire hospital units—stored, maintained, upgraded, and ready to deploy at a moment's notice. Mobile teams trained in rapid assembly and emergency triage can be distributed like a modern medical corps. Countries that invest in such infrastructure transform health security from a passive promise into an active capability.

Critics claim that mobile hospitals are too expensive or too complex to maintain. But the economic calculus of crisis tells a different story. The financial damage caused by delayed response, overwhelmed hospitals, and uncontrolled outbreaks dwarfs the cost of maintaining mobile capacity. Every day of uncontrolled viral spread, every region forced into full lockdown, every collapse of essential services imposes costs measured in billions. By contrast, modular hospitals, once built and standardized, become durable national assets—ready not only for pandemics but for earthquakes, chemical accidents, conflict zones, and climate-driven disasters.

Another critique insists that mobile units can never replace permanent hospitals. But the purpose of mobility is not replacement; it is augmentation. Permanent hospitals remain the backbone of health systems. Mobile capacity becomes the circulatory system that rushes strength to the body's weakest points. Resilience emerges not from static walls but from the ability to move, adapt, and respond.

The century ahead will demand a healthcare system that can bend with the world's volatility. Mobile medicine, combined with AI diagnostics, autonomous logistics, and real-time data streams, offers precisely that. It enables care to reach the crisis rather than waiting for the crisis to reach care. It represents a civilization that has learned not only to treat disease but to anticipate it, surround it, and outmaneuver it.

The Race for Universal Antivirals

If the pandemic response had a central blind spot, it was the overwhelming obsession with vaccines at the expense of antiviral research. Vaccines are indispensable—but they take time, and time is a luxury pandemics do not allow.

The drug Paxlovid demonstrated that the battle against a

virus can also be fought on a biochemical front. By blocking the protease enzyme essential for the SARS-CoV-2 virus to replicate, Paxlovid prevented the infection from spreading within the body. Its dual-component mechanism—nimatrelvir to inhibit viral replication and ritonavir to sustain its concentration—proved to be a model of precision pharmacology.

The lesson is simple: while vaccines prepare the immune system, antivirals act directly on the enemy. And unlike vaccines, they are less vulnerable to viral mutations. The next pandemic may not give the world a year to develop a new vaccine, but a stockpile of broad-spectrum antivirals could be deployed immediately.

Future research must focus on *universal antivirals*—drugs that target the common mechanisms of viral replication rather than the unique features of each strain. Studying the viral life cycle, immune system modulation, and genetic pathways could unlock treatments that apply to entire classes of viruses: coronaviruses, influenza, or even unknown future pathogens.

Investing in virology is not just scientific prudence—it is

existential insurance. The cost of ignorance, as we have learned, is counted in millions of graves and trillions of dollars.

The historical bias toward vaccines becomes even clearer when one recalls their origin. Vaccination began as a response to bacterial killers—smallpox treated through variolation, anthrax through Pasteur's pioneering work, tetanus and diphtheria through the rise of toxoid vaccines. These pathogens were genetically stable, slow to mutate, and biologically predictable. A vaccine developed once could remain effective for decades or even a lifetime. The scientific confidence produced by these early triumphs shaped public-health doctrine for an entire century.

Viruses, however, do not behave like their bacterial predecessors. They evolve with far greater speed, shedding and acquiring mutations with each replication cycle. RNA viruses in particular—coronaviruses, influenza, flaviviruses—operate on an evolutionary fast-forward, rewriting their own blueprints as they spread through populations. A vaccine designed for a bacterial threat could rest on the assumption of biological continuity. A vaccine designed for a viral threat must confront the reality of biological flux.

This discrepancy created a conceptual blind spot. The old model—one pathogen, one vaccine—worked so well for bacteria that it became the default response even to viral diseases. Public health systems inherited this muscle memory. When a new virus appears, global institutions instinctively reach for the vaccine toolkit, even when the virus mutates faster than the research can proceed. The coronavirus illustrated this brutally: by the time vaccine formulations stabilized, new variants were already eroding their precision.

The ease with which viruses evolve is not a peripheral issue; it is the central challenge of modern epidemiology. A pathogen that can reconfigure its antigenic surface forces a perpetual race—one in which humanity must continuously chase yesterday's iteration of the virus. Antivirals break this cycle. They bypass the volatile surface features entirely and strike at the machinery of replication itself, where evolution's room for maneuver is limited by biochemical necessity.

Recognizing this divergence between bacterial stability and viral instability is essential for shaping future strategy. Vaccines remain crucial, but they can no longer be the cornerstone of pandemic response. Their strengths belong to a world where threats were slow and mutations rare. In a world of rapid viral evolution, antivirals must hold equal—if not greater—priority. Only by acknowledging the fundamental differences between bacterial and viral biology can a civilization design defenses worthy of the dangers that lie ahead.

The historical record makes this imbalance unmistakable. For decades, global health policy poured its resources into vaccine platforms while antiviral research proceeded in sporadic bursts—often only after an outbreak had already begun. HIV forced the world to invest in antiretrovirals; hepatitis C pushed research toward polymerase and protease inhibitors; Ebola spurred monoclonal development. Each crisis produced breakthroughs, yet between crises the momentum faded, leaving humanity perpetually unprepared for the next viral assault. Pandemics punish this amnesia with ruthless consistency.

The success of Paxlovid did not emerge from improvisation; it emerged from a foundation of biochemical insight that could—and should—have been built earlier. By targeting a viral protease, the drug exploited a mechanism shared by many RNA viruses. This strategy revealed a larger truth: viruses differ in surface structures, but they converge in the machinery that allows them to hijack the cell. Replication enzymes, entry pathways, nucleic acid synthesis, and protein processing are evolutionary bottlenecks. They cannot mutate freely without destroying the virus itself. These bottlenecks are the universal vulnerabilities of the viral world, and they should be the strategic focus of the next era of pharmacology.

The gap between what was possible and what was pursued became painfully visible when new variants emerged. While vaccines had to be reformulated and redistributed, antivirals retained their potency because they attacked the virus at its core rather than its changing periphery. This resilience should guide scientific priorities. A universal antiviral that inhibits conserved replication pathways would remain effective against a mutating pathogen long after a vaccine's antigen match had decayed. Such drugs could be stockpiled years in advance and deployed the moment an outbreak is detected, containing its spread before exponential growth takes hold.

Modern science already possesses the tools for such breakthroughs. High-throughput screening, cryo-electron microscopy, structure-based drug design, and AI-driven molecular modeling allow researchers to identify conserved viral features with precision unimaginable in past decades. Broad-spectrum candidates exist in early research—polymerase inhibitors that act across multiple virus families, protease inhibitors with cross-viral activity, and host-targeted drugs that block cellular entry rather than viral proteins. These are not distant dreams but underfunded realities awaiting strategic commitment.

A resilient civilization must treat antiviral development as a standing global mission. Nations should maintain permanent research institutes dedicated to viral biochemistry, supported by continuous funding rather than emergency grants. Public–private partnerships can accelerate clinical trials, while international agreements can establish shared antiviral stockpiles, just as some nations already maintain strategic fuel or grain reserves. Manufacturing capacity must be kept warm, not mothballed between crises, ensuring that mass production can begin within days, not months.

Critics may claim that universal antivirals are scientifically unrealistic, pointing to the diversity of viral families. Yet the argument collapses once the focus shifts from surface antigens to conserved enzymatic processes. Viruses vary endlessly in form but remain surprisingly constrained in function. The nature of life itself dictates these constraints; evolution has already done the screening. To exploit these vulnerabilities is not a fantasy but a logical extension of molecular biology.

Others argue that antivirals may encourage resistance. But resistance is not a reason to avoid therapy; it is a reason to design combination treatments, multi-target inhibitors, and rotation protocols—approaches that have already succeeded in HIV and tuberculosis. The tools of resistance management are well established. What is missing is the will to apply them broadly.

The truth is stark and unavoidable. Humanity cannot continue relying on a single defensive pillar. Vaccines are a triumph of science, but they are slow, fragile, and reactive. Antivirals are fast, robust, and proactive. A world that possesses both stands a chance. A world that ignores one will inevitably repeat the tragedies it pretends to regret.

In an age where pathogens travel faster than political decisions, a universal antiviral is not a luxury of research—it is the biochemical equivalent of a fire extinguisher in a world built of dry timber.

A New Economic Contract: Universal Basic Income

Pandemics are not only biological events; they are economic earthquakes. When businesses shutter and entire industries freeze, the vulnerable are always the first to fall. The idea of a *universal basic income* (UBI) has long floated through political discourse as an idealistic dream. The pandemic turned it into a pragmatic necessity.

A UBI would provide every citizen with a financial baseline—a guaranteed income sufficient to cover essential needs, regardless of employment status. During lockdowns, this would have stabilized purchasing power, maintained demand for goods and services, and prevented the spiral of poverty that followed economic shutdowns.

To fund it, a small *microtax* on all financial transactions could suffice: a fraction of a percent on every trade, purchase, or money transfer. Individually negligible, collectively immense. Given the sheer volume of daily financial exchanges, such a system could generate vast public revenue without penalizing workers or small businesses.

This approach would also spread the tax burden evenly across the economic ecosystem, ensuring that corporations and financial institutions contribute proportionally to the public good. In fact, such a mechanism could replace much of the archaic, labyrinthine tax system entirely—simplifying governance while guaranteeing basic social protection.

A universal income, sustained by an automated and transparent system, would not only serve as a safety net in crises but also as a springboard for innovation. People free from existential financial fear could pursue education, entrepreneurship, or creative work. Economic stability would become not a privilege but a right.

The logic of a universal income becomes even clearer when seen through the long arc of economic history. For centuries, societies accepted precarity as a natural condition of life. The industrial age merely formalized this insecurity through wage labor: when the factory closed, the livelihood vanished; when the market failed, entire families were thrown into destitution. Modern capitalism built extraordinary prosperity, but it never resolved its foundational contradiction—its dependence on uninterrupted motion. When that motion stops, even briefly, millions of lives collapse.

The pandemic did not invent this fragility; it exposed it. Within weeks, the global economy revealed its true nature: a structure built on thin margins, household debt, and employment models that assume perpetual stability.

Governments raced to improvise emergency payments, wage subsidies, and stimulus programs—temporary lifeboats for a sinking ship. These measures, though imperfect, revealed a profound truth: when states choose to act decisively, poverty is not an inevitability but a policy choice.

A universal basic income transforms this insight into a permanent architecture. Instead of sporadic rescue packages, society gains a continuous stabilizer. When crises arrive—pandemics, recessions, climate disasters—the financial floor does not shatter. Consumers maintain purchasing power, businesses retain customers, and economic contraction slows instead of cascading into freefall. UBI becomes not a welfare mechanism but a macroeconomic safety valve.

The microtax model makes this stabilization self-sustaining. Every transaction—whether executed by an individual, a corporation, or an algorithmic trading system—contributes an infinitesimal amount to the social foundation. The burden becomes proportional to activity rather than income, aligning taxation with the true velocity of modern economies. In a world where trillions move through digital channels daily, even a microscopic levy generates revenue far beyond what conventional taxation can reliably collect.

Such a system also accomplishes something the current tax architecture struggles to achieve: universality. Wealth generated by high-frequency financial activity, multinational operations, and automated trading no longer escapes national borders through loopholes or relocations. It contributes automatically, in real time, without the need for audits, enforcement campaigns, or decades-long political battles. Taxation becomes a property of the financial system itself, as intrinsic as gravity in physics.

The social consequences of such reform extend far beyond crisis response. When basic survival is guaranteed, the economy becomes more innovative, not less. People take calculated risks because failure no longer threatens starvation. Education becomes purposeful rather than desperate. Creativity flourishes when fear recedes. A society where citizens have the freedom to choose their paths produces scientific breakthroughs, artistic movements, and entrepreneurial revolutions that rigid survival-based systems cannot replicate.

Critics warn that universal income may disincentivize work. But evidence from pilot programs tells a different story. When freed from existential anxiety, people tend to work more productively and pursue higher-value tasks rather than low-wage drudgery. The disappearance of extreme poverty does not create idleness; it creates possibility. Work becomes chosen rather than coerced, and economies built on choice perform better than those built on compulsion.

The deeper argument is civilizational. A world entering an era of automation, pandemics, and environmental volatility cannot rely on nineteenth-century economic logic. Machine labor will increasingly outperform human labor in routine tasks; entire industries will transform faster than political institutions can adapt. A universal basic income offers stability in a future defined by disruption. It is not charity but infrastructure—the economic equivalent of clean water or electricity.

A society that guarantees every person a baseline of

dignity builds resilience not just against pandemics but against every form of turbulence the coming century will deliver. In such a world, security is no longer the privilege of the lucky; it becomes the birthright of the human species.

The rise of artificial intelligence, robotics, and full-scale automation only intensifies this necessity. Long before the next pandemic arrives, the world will face an economic transformation far more profound than any previous technological shift. Machines are no longer limited to physical labor; they now perform cognitive tasks once believed to be the exclusive domain of human intelligence. Algorithms trade securities, diagnose diseases, negotiate logistics, generate legal drafts, write code, and create art. Robots assemble products with flawless precision, coordinate warehouses without fatigue, and perform maintenance in environments where human labor is expensive, dangerous, or unnecessary.

This is not a future threat—it is a present reality accelerating with each passing year. As automation advances, entire sectors will be reshaped. Routine administrative roles, basic manufacturing jobs, transportation work, and clerical positions will diminish. Even white-collar professions will not remain untouched; the boundary between "skilled" and "automatable" is dissolving. An economy built on employment as the primary conduit of income cannot survive a world where machines outperform humans at scale.

A universal basic income becomes the stabilizing framework for this new age. It absorbs the shock of rapid automation, ensuring that prosperity does not vanish into the hands of those who own the algorithms while the majority face economic dislocation. It converts technological progress into shared progress, allowing society to benefit from automation rather than suffer from it.

A microtax on automated transactions aligns perfectly with this transformation. As machine-driven systems come to dominate financial markets, logistics, and productivity networks, the flow of value becomes increasingly digital. Taxation tied to human labor becomes obsolete. Taxation tied to the velocity of automated economic activity becomes both fair and efficient. It captures revenue precisely where value is generated—in the constant motion of digital capital and algorithmic exchange.

In such a system, the wealth created by automation is reinvested into the society whose stability makes that automation possible. Productivity gains are no longer hoarded but distributed. Innovation is no longer feared but welcomed. A person whose income is not tied to the volatility of the labor market can navigate the future with agency rather than anxiety. The fear that automation will make millions economically obsolete evaporates once society guarantees that the benefits of automation flow back to the people themselves.

The alternative is a world divided sharply between those who own the machines and those replaced by them. Such a civilization would be unstable, prone to political upheaval, social fragmentation, and economic insecurity. But with a universal basic income anchored to an automatic, technology-driven tax base, automation becomes not a threat to employment but a liberation from drudgery. Human creativity, care, imagination, and innovation become central to the new economy, while machines carry the burden of routine work.

This convergence of AI, automation, and economic reform is not a matter of ideology; it is a matter of survival. The same technological forces that transform society threaten to destabilize it unless the economic contract is rewritten. A universal income ensures that progress does not destroy the human beings it was meant to uplift. It transforms automation into a civilizational advantage rather than a destabilizing force. It ensures that humanity enters the age of intelligent machines with dignity, security, and purpose intact.

The Global Mind: Data, Science, and Cooperation

No nation can fight a pandemic alone. Viruses recognize no borders, and ignorance in one country can ignite disaster in another. What humanity needs is an *international digital immune system*: a platform for the rapid, secure exchange of data on emerging pathogens, mutations, treatments, and clinical outcomes.

Such a system would function as a shared intelligence hub. When a new virus is detected, its genetic sequence, epidemiological data, and clinical characteristics should be uploaded instantly, accessible to researchers worldwide. This would allow scientists to begin vaccine and drug development within days, not months.

Standardized data formats, blockchain verification, and AI-driven analytics could ensure transparency and reliability. This network could also coordinate clinical trials, share findings, and prevent redundant research—accelerating discovery while conserving resources.

Naturally, information security must be paramount. The system must protect privacy and prevent misuse. But secrecy and nationalism in the face of a global threat are luxuries humanity can no longer afford. The next pandemic will demand global coordination at a speed and scale we have never achieved before.

The foundations of such a global system already exist in

fragmented form. Platforms like GISAID, which collected and shared viral genetic sequences during COVID-19, proved how transformative rapid information exchange can be. Within days of the first reported cases, scientists sequenced the virus and made the data publicly available, enabling laboratories across continents to begin designing diagnostics and early vaccine prototypes. This unprecedented openness saved countless lives. Yet even GISAID functioned as a voluntary consortium rather than an integrated global infrastructure. Data arrived in uneven waves; some nations contributed fully, others partially, and some withheld information entirely. The result was a patchwork of cooperation in a world that required seamless unity.

To evolve from patchwork to architecture, global health intelligence must be conceived as a planetary commons— an institution with the same inevitability as international air traffic control or maritime safety conventions. Just as airplanes rely on shared skies, science must rely on shared data. Under such a system, every nation becomes a sentinel node in a global network, contributing its insights and receiving the world's insights in return. No single country bears the burden of surveillance alone; responsibility is distributed, and benefits are collective.

The scientific acceleration produced by true data integration would be extraordinary. AI-driven modeling could track the early dynamics of an outbreak with unprecedented precision, identifying hotspots before they ignite into uncontrolled spread. Mutation monitoring would become continuous, allowing researchers to detect dangerous variants the moment they arise rather than months later. Clinical feedback loops would shorten from years to weeks: treatment protocols that show promise in one region could be tested, validated, and adapted in others almost immediately. This is the difference between fighting a global enemy with scattered militias or with a coordinated intelligence force.

While global cooperation is valuable, the reforms proposed in this book do not depend on it. Every element of the architecture—cluster-based settlement, autonomous logistics, modular healthcare, unified national data systems, and automated supply infrastructure—can be implemented entirely within the borders of a single country. A nation that restructures its internal systems becomes resilient regardless of whether others follow. International exchanges may accelerate research, but they are not prerequisites for survival. The essential insight is that preparedness is fundamentally local: every country must be capable of functioning during global disruption, even when borders close and international coordination falters.

Of course, global cooperation demands trust, and trust demands safeguards. Data privacy, national sovereignty, and cybersecurity cannot be afterthoughts; they must be embedded into the system's architecture. Cryptographic verification ensures that data cannot be altered. Decentralized storage prevents any single actor from controlling or manipulating information. And differential privacy techniques allow sensitive clinical data to contribute to global insight without revealing personal identities. Security becomes a feature, not a compromise.

However, the greater danger lies not in openness but in isolation. When nations hide outbreaks, suppress data, or delay reporting, the consequences ripple far beyond their borders. The coronavirus taught this brutally: delayed transparency in one region gave the virus a head start across the entire world. A global immune system prevents such failures by replacing secrecy with structured obligation and replacing suspicion with verified cooperation.

This vision is not only a scientific necessity but a moral one. Humanity's adversaries—viruses, climate disruptions, economic shocks—are indifferent to passports and borders. They exploit human division as readily as biological weakness. A species that shares the same vulnerabilities must share the same intelligence. Only a unified global mind can protect eight billion bodies.

The next pandemic will not test the strength of individual nations; it will test the connectedness of civilization itself. The societies that embrace knowledge-sharing as instinct rather than negotiation will form the first line of defense for all humankind.

The Psychology of Calm

Finally, one of the most underestimated aspects of crisis management is psychological stability. Panic can cripple societies faster than any pathogen. The constant churn of sensational media, the barrage of contradictory statements from officials, and the politicization of science all serve to erode public trust.

The architecture proposed in this book does not rely on social trust. It is designed precisely to function in societies where trust is low, institutions are fragile, and public confidence fluctuates. Trust is a sociological variable, but autonomous logistics, modular housing, unified medical databases, and distributed supply chains are engineering constants. A drone does not require public reassurance to deliver insulin. A modular cluster does not depend on political culture to remain self-sufficient. A national medical system does not degrade because citizens distrust government statements. The purpose of this architecture is to remove trust as a prerequisite for stability. When systems are built to operate automatically and locally, psychological cohesion becomes optional, not foundational. Preparedness should not be a moral mood— it should be a property of infrastructure.

What we need in future crises is not more drama, but more clarity. Authorities must communicate calmly, transparently, and consistently—informing rather than frightening. Every policy must be justified by evidence, not theater. Instead of blanket restrictions imposed for optics, focus should be placed on precision measures: isolating clusters, enhancing testing, and protecting the vulnerable.

The media, too, bears responsibility. Information should illuminate, not inflame. Fear is contagious, but so is reason.

Mass panic is not a natural force that erupts from human psychology; it is an engineered outcome of an information environment that rewards fear, outrage, and sensationalism. The hysteria surrounding COVID-19 did not arise from the public but from a media ecosystem that broadcast danger twenty-four hours a day, magnifying every uncertainty into catastrophe and every anomaly into existential threat. People did not lose their minds spontaneously; they were overwhelmed by a continuous stream of fear signals designed for attention economics. The book does not claim that technology eliminates human emotions. It argues that emotions cease to destabilize society when they are no longer amplified by an information system that treats anxiety as a commodity. Preparedness is not a psychological cure—it is the removal of the megaphone that turns ordinary concern into mass hysteria.

A society's psychological equilibrium is itself a form of infrastructure. When fear becomes unregulated, it spreads through populations with the same exponential velocity as a virus, overwhelming judgment, distorting perception, and driving people toward behaviors that worsen the crisis. Panic buying, conspiracy spirals, mass distrust of institutions, refusal of medical care, and social fragmentation are not biological phenomena; they are cognitive breakdowns triggered when citizens no longer believe the information they receive.

The pandemic revealed how fragile collective psychology

truly is. Inconsistent messaging—whether about masks, transmission, vaccines, or lockdowns—created cognitive dissonance that the public interpreted as deception. When officials shifted positions without explaining the underlying science, the shifts were read not as adaptation but as incompetence. In this vacuum of trust, misinformation flourished, filling the gaps left by poor communication. This dynamic repeated across nations regardless of political orientation, proving that the weakness was structural, not ideological.

Calm, coordinated messaging is not a luxury; it is a strategic necessity. A population that understands the rationale behind measures complies more willingly than one that feels manipulated. Transparent explanations generate resilience: even difficult policies, when honestly communicated, are met with far greater acceptance than paternalistic directives issued without justification. The psychological immune system of a nation depends on the belief that its leaders are speaking plainly and with integrity.

Precision matters as well. When measures are narrow,

targeted, and evidence-driven, people perceive them as rational rather than punitive. Targeted testing, cluster isolation, and rapid containment strategies preserve normal life for the majority while addressing real risks for the minority. These approaches reduce the psychological fatigue that accumulates under broad, indefinite restrictions. A population whose daily life remains mostly intact sustains discipline longer and avoids the burnout that leads to noncompliance.

The media's role in sustaining psychological stability cannot be overstated. Sensationalism may drive clicks, but it corrodes collective resilience. Information must distinguish between caution and alarm, between seriousness and hysteria. Responsible reporting treats citizens as thinking adults, not emotional targets. Media that prioritizes clarity over shock becomes part of the solution rather than part of the contagion.

Yet the public also carries responsibility. Citizens must cultivate informational hygiene, learning to question sources, verify claims, and resist the emotional lure of outrage. A psychologically mature society does not demand perfection from its institutions but seeks coherence, transparency, and shared purpose.

The psychology of calm, therefore, is not passive. It is an active discipline—a civic virtue woven into the fabric of crisis response. When leaders communicate with honesty, when institutions avoid theatrics, when media reports responsibly, and when individuals cultivate critical thinking, panic finds no oxygen. Society becomes less reactive and more deliberate, transforming fear into informed vigilance.

In the crises ahead—pandemic, climatic, economic, or geopolitical—the capacity for calm will be as essential as any vaccine, antiviral, or technological innovation. It is the psychological shield that allows civilization to think clearly in the presence of danger.

If there is one truth that unites all these lessons, it is this: humanity cannot afford to stumble into the next catastrophe with the same arrogance and confusion that defined the last. The tools of survival are already in our hands—technology, cooperation, and foresight.

The only question that remains is whether we will use them before it is too late.

CHAPTER 3. THE RATIONAL RESPONSE: SCIENCE, CALM, AND COMPASSION IN CRISIS

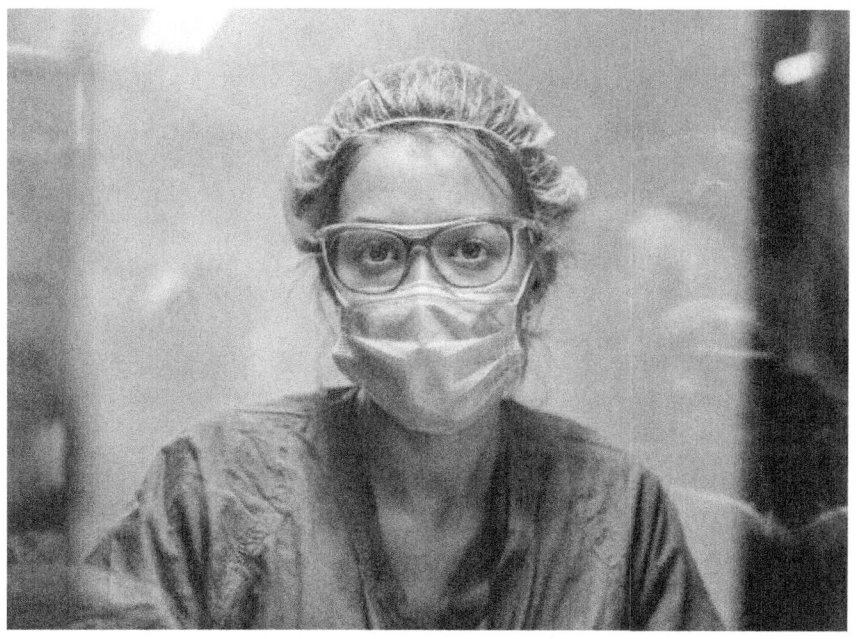

If there is one enduring lesson from the COVID-19 pandemic, it is that panic and politics are as deadly as pathogens. The world didn't just battle a virus—it battled noise. Every television screen and smartphone became a transmitter of hysteria, while governments scrambled to project competence through performance rather than through results. Amid the clamor, science often spoke softly, drowned out by sensationalism and partisanship.

A prudent approach to a pandemic must be rooted in reason. Measures should be taken not because they look decisive, but because data and evidence say they work. Communication with the public must be calm, consistent, and transparent. Nothing breeds panic faster than confusion, and nothing restores trust faster than honesty. People can endure great hardship if they understand *why*—but when they sense deception or incompetence, they rebel.

Had COVID-19 been handled without political posturing, media hysteria, and ideological division, its trajectory could have been far less devastating. Without the constant drama, fewer people would have succumbed to fear; fewer decisions would have been driven by optics rather than necessity. A society that trusts its institutions behaves rationally—and rational behavior is the cornerstone of effective disease control.

Less polarization would have meant less resistance to protective measures. Masks, vaccines, and lockdowns would not have become symbols of political allegiance. The conversation would have shifted from "who's right" to "what works." Cooperation between nations could have replaced competition for vaccines and medical supplies. Instead of exploiting the crisis for political advantage, countries might have shared expertise, data, and resources—saving lives rather than headlines.

Without the constant spectacle of showmanship and scapegoating, governments could have focused on the mechanics of response: accelerating research, streamlining testing, coordinating logistics, and ensuring timely treatment. The pandemic could have become a challenge of intelligent collaboration, not a battlefield of egos. The losses—both human and economic—would have been drastically lower.

Balancing Prevention and Treatment

Vaccines were the crown jewel of the pandemic response, but they were not a panacea. The rush to develop and distribute them overshadowed another vital front: treatment. Pandemics are not merely battles to *prevent* disease, but also to *mitigate* it once it appears.

Developing antiviral drugs that target viral replication and inflammation should have been an equal priority. Drugs like Paxlovid demonstrated that effective treatment can dramatically reduce the severity of infection and mortality rates, especially when administered early. Paxlovid's mechanism—blocking the protease enzyme essential for the SARS-CoV-2 virus to reproduce—represents a paradigm shift: treating the disease at its biochemical roots rather than just stimulating the immune system to defend against it.

Unlike vaccines, which require months or years of development and adaptation to new mutations, antivirals can be deployed immediately once infection begins. Their effectiveness does not depend on predicting the next variant; it depends on targeting the virus's universal survival machinery. In that sense, antivirals are not reactive but inherently adaptive.

The tragedy of COVID-19 was not only the virus itself, but the delay in making such drugs widely available. Bureaucratic inertia, uneven distribution, and rigid approval processes meant that many people died waiting for treatments that already existed. Had antiviral therapies been prioritized alongside vaccines, the global death toll might have been vastly reduced.

The imbalance between prevention and treatment reflects a deeper flaw in global health strategy: a fixation on singular solutions rather than multipronged resilience. The twentieth century taught institutions to view vaccines as the ultimate triumph of medical science—a tool that eliminated smallpox, controlled polio, and pushed numerous childhood diseases into retreat. But this success created an illusion that the immune system alone could be trained to outpace every threat. Viral evolution shattered that illusion. The pandemic made clear that a civilization cannot rely on immune preparation while neglecting the pharmacological tools needed to combat infection once prevention fails.

Treatment has always been the forgotten half of pandemic defense. Historically, antiviral development lags decades behind vaccine innovation, not because antivirals are less important, but because they are scientifically more demanding and economically less glamorous. Vaccines promise eradication; antivirals promise management. Yet it is management—not eradication—that determines survival during the first critical months of an outbreak. An antiviral administered within the first days of infection can prevent hospitalization, reduce viral load, and halt transmission chains before they become unmanageable. A vaccine, no matter how effective, cannot help those already infected.

The necessity of balancing these two pillars becomes even clearer when examining the evolutionary dynamics of viruses. A pathogen confronted only with vaccine-induced immunity will mutate toward immune escape, especially when transmission remains high. But a pathogen confronted with antivirals that attack conserved replication mechanisms faces far fewer evolutionary pathways

The Importance of Early and Comprehensive Care

Effective pandemic management isn't limited to vaccines

and antivirals—it also requires intelligent clinical strategy. During COVID-19, isolation policies, while necessary for containment, often condemned patients to solitude when they most needed care. Many mild cases escalated into critical conditions because people were left untreated until it was too late.

One of the key lessons is the importance of identifying and addressing *secondary bacterial infections*. Viral illnesses such as COVID-19 weaken the immune system, leaving patients vulnerable to bacterial pneumonia and other complications. Ironically, many who died "of COVID" may have actually succumbed to bacterial infections that could have been prevented with timely antibiotic intervention.

Medical staff in isolation wards or telemedicine networks must have access to rapid diagnostic tools that can detect these complications early. The integration of home-monitoring systems, wearable sensors, and remote consultation platforms could enable real-time evaluation of symptoms and prompt treatment before the patient deteriorates.

Prevention of severe complications should also include maintaining oxygen saturation, hydration, and lung health through noninvasive treatments such as oxygen therapy or CPAP devices. Every escalation avoided means one less ventilator needed—and countless lives saved.

In future pandemics, treatment strategies must evolve from reactive crisis management to proactive patient support. Every delay costs lives; every unnecessary isolation without oversight is a silent tragedy.

The tragedy of delayed care was not the fault of medicine, but of systems built around outdated assumptions. At the start of the pandemic, clinical models treated COVID-19 as a purely viral pneumonia, overlooking the complex cascade of immunological and bacterial interactions it triggered. Hospitals prepared for ventilators, but the real battle unfolded much earlier—in bedrooms, apartments, and isolation rooms where patients deteriorated unseen. Medicine had the tools; the infrastructure did not.

Early comprehensive care must therefore become a foundational principle of future pandemic response. The evidence is unequivocal: most patients do not crash suddenly. They decline gradually, through identifiable physiological markers—rising inflammatory proteins, falling oxygen saturation, changes in respiratory pattern, or the onset of bacterial co-infection. The catastrophe of 2020 was that these indicators were often noticed only when patients arrived gasping at emergency rooms, already hours or days beyond the optimal treatment window.

A modernized clinical strategy must close this gap. Continuous monitoring should begin the moment a patient tests positive, not when they arrive at the hospital doorstep. Home-based diagnostic kits capable of measuring CRP, D-dimer, procalcitonin, and oxygen saturation would allow physicians to detect early warning signs of bacterial pneumonia, microclotting, or silent hypoxia long before visible symptoms appear. Wearable sensors already exist that track respiratory rate, coughing frequency, and heart-rate variability with remarkable precision—metrics that often change before subjective symptoms do.

Integrating these tools into telemedicine networks

transforms the patient experience. Instead of isolation becoming abandonment, isolation becomes supervised recovery. Physicians can intervene the moment complications arise, prescribing antibiotics when bacterial infection is confirmed, initiating anti-inflammatory protocols when immune overactivation threatens, or delivering portable oxygen concentrators before saturation levels plunge. This proactive model shifts the locus of care from crisis rooms to living rooms, preventing countless unnecessary hospitalizations.

Lung support is equally crucial. Noninvasive ventilation—CPAP, BiPAP, or high-flow nasal oxygen—was underutilized in early COVID response due to fears of aerosolization, fears later shown to be exaggerated when proper filtration was used. These tools stabilize patients without the risks of intubation, buying time for antivirals and antibiotics to take effect. Widespread access to such devices, supported by telemedical oversight, can prevent the dangerous cascade from mild disease to respiratory collapse.

Crucially, this vision aligns with the nature of pandemics

themselves. Pathogens do not wait for hospital beds to become available, and health systems cannot scale infinitely. But early, distributed, intelligent care reduces the burden on hospitals by preventing deterioration in the first place. The most advanced healthcare systems in the world fail when they are saturated; the most modest systems succeed when patients never require intensive care.

The shift from reactive to proactive medicine requires investment not only in equipment but in architecture: home-delivery networks for pharmaceuticals and oxygen, diagnostic algorithms that triage risk in real time, and clinical protocols designed for early intervention rather than late rescue. It also demands reform in communication. Patients must be educated—calmly and clearly—about warning signs, the importance of monitoring, and the availability of remote support. Fear drives people to hide symptoms; knowledge drives them to seek help early.

What emerges is a philosophy of care that respects both biology and humanity. Illness need not mean abandonment; quarantine need not mean solitary suffering. When societies design their medical systems around early detection, continuous support, and humane oversight, pandemics become less lethal not through dramatic heroics, but through steady, intelligent stewardship.

A future in which no one dies alone, unseen, or untreated is not a utopian dream. It is the logical next step for a civilization that chooses foresight over improvisation, compassion over panic, and knowledge over passive waiting.

Antibiotics and the Forgotten Battle

One of the most overlooked realities of the pandemic is that many patients did not die from the virus itself. They died from bacterial pneumonia, sepsis, and other secondary infections that exploited weakened immune systems. Yet the global discourse focused almost exclusively on viral transmission, masking the importance of early antibiotic use in high-risk patients.

This neglect was partly ideological: public messaging against antibiotic misuse was so strong that, in the pandemic's chaos, the pendulum swung too far in the opposite direction. Doctors hesitated to prescribe them even when clinically justified. As a result, treatable bacterial infections often went unchecked until they became fatal.

A balanced policy is essential. While antibiotic stewardship remains critical to preventing resistance, a blanket aversion to their use during viral pandemics is equally dangerous. Clear clinical guidelines should define when and how to administer antibiotics as prophylaxis against bacterial complications in severe viral cases.

Future pandemic strategies must include education and training for healthcare professionals on this issue, ensuring that the war against one pathogen does not blind us to another.

The oversight surrounding antibiotics during the pandemic revealed a paradox at the heart of modern medicine. After decades of warnings about antibiotic resistance, clinical culture became so cautious that even justified use was viewed with suspicion. Public health messaging, though well-intentioned, conflated stewardship with avoidance, creating an atmosphere in which the fear of contributing to resistance overshadowed the immediate need to save lives. This shift did not emerge overnight—it was the culmination of years in which antibiotics were framed primarily as a threat rather than a tool, and this framing left clinicians psychologically unprepared for a crisis in which bacterial opportunists became as deadly as the virus itself.

Historical memory should have guided policy. Every major influenza pandemic—including the 1918 catastrophe—demonstrated that secondary bacterial pneumonia is often the true killer. Autopsy studies from past outbreaks consistently found streptococcal and staphylococcal infections as the final cause of death. The same pattern reappeared in COVID-19: the virus opened the door, and bacteria walked through it. Yet this well-documented reality was largely ignored in the early strategic discourse, which focused almost exclusively on viral dynamics while overlooking the microbial ecosystem that evolves in the wake of viral damage.

The biological mechanisms are straightforward. Viral infections disrupt the epithelial barriers of the respiratory tract, impair mucociliary clearance, and weaken immune surveillance. In this compromised environment, bacteria that ordinarily coexist harmlessly within the nasopharyngeal flora can invade deeper tissues, causing pneumonia that escalates rapidly without early intervention. Once bacterial sepsis sets in, survival becomes a race against time—one that cannot be won without immediate antibiotic therapy.

A modern pandemic response must therefore integrate bacterial defense into its core architecture. Clinical pathways should include standardized criteria for initiating antibiotics in high-risk viral patients—those with comorbidities, radiographic evidence of bacterial involvement, elevated inflammatory markers suggestive of coinfection, or rapid clinical deterioration. Rapid diagnostic technologies, such as multiplex PCR panels and procalcitonin measurement, can distinguish viral disease from bacterial superinfection within hours rather than days, reducing uncertainty and guiding precise treatment rather than blind overuse.

Antibiotic stewardship should not be abandoned—it must be refined. Stewardship does not mean withholding antibiotics reflexively; it means using them intelligently. In pandemics, intelligent use requires flexible, evidence-based protocols that adapt to the dynamic interplay between viruses and bacteria. Stewardship committees should operate alongside emergency response teams to ensure that life-saving antibiotics are deployed swiftly where needed and avoided where unnecessary.

Education is equally vital. Many healthcare professionals entered the pandemic with strong anti-antibiotic biases shaped by years of public messaging. Training must recalibrate this mindset, teaching clinicians how to recognize early signs of bacterial invasion, how to balance risks, and how to integrate antibiotics into a holistic approach that includes antivirals, anti-inflammatories, and supportive care. Clear national guidelines, widely disseminated and regularly updated, can prevent the confusion and hesitation that cost so many lives.

The deeper lesson is that pandemics do not occur in microbial isolation. They are ecological events that destabilize the entire microbial environment of the human body. Ignoring bacterial opportunists in a viral storm is as dangerous as ignoring embers in a forest fire. The next pandemic will demand vigilance on all fronts—viral, bacterial, and systemic. A balanced, evidence-driven antibiotic strategy is not a footnote to viral response; it is one of its essential pillars.

Rethinking Vaccine Prioritization

Vaccination remains one of humanity's most powerful tools against infectious disease—but its effectiveness depends on strategy, not just science. During the pandemic, chaotic rollout plans and inconsistent messaging undermined trust and efficiency.

A rational vaccination policy must prioritize the

vulnerable and the essential. The elderly, chronically ill, and immunocompromised must come first, as they face the highest risk of severe outcomes. Next are healthcare workers, first responders, and public service personnel—those whose health sustains the very infrastructure of society.

Logistics are as critical as biology. Mobile vaccination units, decentralized distribution centers, and drone-assisted delivery can ensure that even remote or immobile populations receive timely access. Transparent communication about vaccine safety, necessity, and prioritization can dispel misinformation and build public confidence.

Vaccination should never be treated as a political spectacle or a moral referendum—it is a public health operation. Its goal is protection, not propaganda.

Yet effective vaccination strategy requires more than a clear sequence of priority groups; it demands a philosophy of deployment rooted in epidemiological logic rather than political theatrics. The early months of COVID-19 showed how easily public trust can be fractured when vaccination becomes entangled with national pride, ideological battles, or competitive posturing between political factions. Vaccines, when framed as symbols of loyalty or conformity, lose the neutrality essential to public health. A successful campaign must therefore remove vaccination from the arena of identity and return it to the domain of strategy.

The core of that strategy is to reduce mortality first, then transmission, then disruption. This sequence is not ideological but mathematical. Protecting the highest-risk individuals decreases deaths. Protecting essential workers preserves the functioning of hospitals, transportation, utilities, governance, and food supply chains. Immunizing high-contact populations—teachers, service workers, public transportation staff—reduces community spread. When these layers align, society gains stability, and fear gives way to predictability.

But prioritization fails without access. In the last pandemic, urban centers received doses rapidly while rural communities waited, and marginalized populations—those with limited mobility, limited technology, or limited trust in institutions—were often the last to be reached. A resilient system cannot rely on static clinics or the assumption that citizens will travel long distances to receive care. Vaccination must move toward people, not the other way around. Mobile units, pop-up clinics in community centers and schools, neighborhood outreach teams, and drone delivery for remote areas convert vaccination from a passive offering into an active service.

Equally important is the architecture of information. Misinformation thrives where governments communicate vaguely, inconsistently, or condescendingly. A vaccination policy that explains its logic openly—why certain groups come first, how safety is monitored, what side effects are expected, and how long immunity may last—creates a psychological environment where trust grows rather than erodes. Transparency is not an optional courtesy; it is a strategic tool for achieving compliance without coercion.

The global experience also revealed that vaccine hesitancy is not a monolith. Some resist because they distrust institutions; others because they fear side effects; others because they feel overlooked or disrespected by the systems meant to protect them. Addressing these concerns requires communication tailored to communities rather than one-size-fits-all messaging. Faith leaders, local physicians, community organizers, and culturally informed outreach teams can convey information with authority that centralized broadcasts often fail to command.

Finally, vaccine strategy must be dynamic. Variant emergence may require updated formulations, booster schedules, or targeted micro-campaigns in high-risk zones. A rigid plan becomes obsolete as soon as the virus evolves; a flexible plan evolves alongside it. Future vaccination systems must therefore be designed as adaptable networks, capable of shifting supply lines, recalibrating priorities, and integrating new data without bureaucratic delay.

What emerges is a vision of vaccination as a disciplined operation rather than a symbolic act—an intervention guided by evidence, logistics, and clarity. When vaccines are deployed intelligently, they become a stabilizing force; when they are deployed chaotically, they become a source of confusion and division. The difference lies not in the science of the vaccine itself, but in the wisdom of the society that administers it.

The Hidden Toll: Collateral Deaths and Neglected Patients

Perhaps the most haunting aspect of the pandemic was the silent suffering of those who were not infected at all. Hospitals overwhelmed by COVID-19 cases turned away patients with cancer, heart disease, and other chronic conditions. Elective surgeries were postponed indefinitely; diagnostic screenings vanished from schedules.

Millions lost access to essential care, leading to surges in deaths from non-COVID causes. People with chest pain avoided hospitals out of fear of infection. Diabetics missed checkups. Cancer patients skipped chemotherapy.

Entire branches of medicine went dark in the shadow of a single disease.

The irony is cruel: in the rush to save lives from the virus, the world neglected countless others. Mental health also buckled under the weight of isolation, fear, and economic collapse. Depression, anxiety, and suicide rates soared. For some, the "cure" was worse than the disease.

The next pandemic must be fought on *two fronts*: the biological and the social. Healthcare systems must maintain parallel capacity for routine and emergency care. Telemedicine, digital triage, and home diagnostics can ensure continuity of treatment even in lockdown conditions. Neglecting the non-pandemic patient is not strategy—it is surrender.

The collateral deaths of the pandemic were not inevitable; they were the consequence of a brittle healthcare architecture designed for ordinary times and incapable of walking and chewing gum simultaneously. For decades, hospital systems across the world operated on thin margins—just enough beds, just enough staff, just enough equipment to handle predictable demands. This "efficiency" collapsed the moment unpredictability arrived. When COVID-19 surged, the entire system bent toward a single priority, revealing a structural blindness: the assumption that crises occur in isolation.

History has warned of this before. During the 2014 West African Ebola outbreak, deaths from malaria, tuberculosis, and childbirth complications skyrocketed— not because treatments ceased to exist, but because the machinery of care was paralyzed. The same pattern reappeared in 2020. Health systems that dedicated themselves exclusively to the pandemic inadvertently created a shadow pandemic of neglected disease. Excess mortality analyses from multiple countries later revealed that a significant portion of deaths occurred not from COVID itself, but from the vacuum of care left in its wake.

The psychological dimension deepened this toll. Fear became a deterrent strong enough to override chest pain, stroke symptoms, or signs of advancing infection. People stayed home when they should have sought help, and by the time they finally arrived, conditions that were treatable days earlier had turned irreversible. The very places designed to heal became perceived as dangerous, not because of their function but because of their failure to communicate safety and maintain continuity.

A resilient healthcare system must therefore possess bifurcation capacity: the ability to expand pandemic response without collapsing routine medical care. This requires prebuilt redundancy—parallel care pathways, dedicated "clean" hospitals or wings, and telehealth scaffolding capable of absorbing routine consultations without forcing patients into crowded facilities. Digital triage can transform primary care by directing patients to appropriate services without clogging emergency rooms. Remote monitoring for chronic illnesses—glucose sensors, cardiac telemetry, virtual oncology check-ins—allows treatment continuity without physical exposure.

Specialty medicine must be shielded as well. Cancer units, dialysis centers, maternity wards, and emergency cardiac services should operate under separate operational protocols during crises, with autonomous supply chains and staffing pools. These are not luxuries; they are lifelines. The shutdown of such essential services in 2020 created delayed waves of tragedy, visible only months later when late-stage diagnoses surged and preventable deaths multiplied.

Mental health requires equal attention. Isolation policies, though epidemiologically justified, carried deep psychological costs. A society cannot preserve biological life while disregarding emotional life. Crisis response must integrate mental health hotlines, virtual counseling, and community support networks from the outset. Lockdowns without psychological infrastructure become pressure cookers; lockdowns with support become manageable protective measures.

Critics argue that building parallel capacity is too expensive. But the economic burden of untreated chronic disease—lost productivity, long-term disability, emergency interventions—far outweighs the investment required to keep essential care running. A society that shuts down healthcare to fight a virus merely shifts the burden to future months in the form of delayed catastrophe.

The lesson is stark: a pandemic is never a single battle. It is a war on multiple fronts—viral, psychological, social, and chronic. To prioritize one front while abandoning the others is not strategy; it is tunnel vision. A truly prepared civilization maintains the health of all its citizens, not just those caught in the spotlight of the latest pathogen.

The Mental Health Imperative

No crisis is purely physical. Pandemics strike at the mind as much as the body. The isolation, uncertainty, and economic precarity of COVID-19 left millions psychologically scarred. Yet mental health services were often the first to collapse under restrictions.

Digital technology offers a solution. Online platforms can provide psychological support when physical presence is impossible. Virtual counseling, group therapy sessions, and self-help programs can be made accessible through secure, user-friendly systems. These services should be multilingual, inclusive, and available across age groups—from teenagers paralyzed by anxiety to the elderly grappling with loneliness.

Governments must treat mental health not as an afterthought but as an integral part of public health planning. Just as we stockpile masks and ventilators, we should invest in mental resilience—training counselors, developing digital infrastructure, and destigmatizing psychological care.

A population that is calm, informed, and emotionally supported is far more resilient than one ruled by fear.

The psychological devastation of the pandemic revealed an uncomfortable truth: mental health is not a peripheral concern but a core determinant of national stability. Fear alters cognition. Isolation erodes emotional regulation. Economic insecurity magnifies despair. A population under psychological siege becomes harder to govern, harder to educate, harder to heal. When the mind collapses, the body follows. And yet, in the early months of the pandemic, mental health infrastructure evaporated almost overnight—not because the need diminished, but because the systems designed to support it were fragile, centralized, and tied to physical presence.

The invisibility of psychological suffering made it easier for governments to overlook. Hospital wards filled with COVID patients provided stark images that dominated headlines, while the quiet despair in living rooms, dormitories, and long-term care homes remained largely unseen. But the statistical record eventually revealed the magnitude of the damage: spikes in anxiety disorders, depressive episodes, substance abuse, domestic violence, and suicide attempts. These second-order tragedies did not appear as dramatic curves on epidemiological charts, yet they shaped the lived experience of millions far more profoundly than the virus itself.

A resilient society must therefore build a mental health architecture as robust as its medical one. Digital tools provide the foundation for such a transformation. Virtual counseling eliminates barriers of distance, stigma, and mobility; it can reach communities where psychiatrists and therapists are scarce. Online group therapy restores a sense of belonging to those cut off from social contact. AI-assisted triage systems can identify individuals at high risk of crisis and direct them to appropriate services. Secure digital platforms allow continuity of care even when physical clinics close.

But technology alone is insufficient. A psychological care system must be woven into the fabric of crisis planning. Governments should maintain protected mental health budgets that do not evaporate during emergencies. Schools need protocols for supporting children during prolonged closures, incorporating virtual socialization, structured routines, and counseling access. Workplaces must adopt mental health safeguards for employees facing rapid transitions, uncertainty, or isolation. Elderly populations require targeted interventions to prevent loneliness from escalating into cognitive decline or clinical depression.

Destigmatization is equally crucial. Many suffer silently not because help is unavailable, but because they fear judgment or dismissal. Public messaging must normalize psychological distress during crises, framing therapy as a tool of strength rather than weakness. Community leaders, educators, and healthcare workers should be trained to recognize early signs of mental strain and direct individuals toward appropriate resources before their suffering becomes acute.

Preparedness also demands redundancy. Just as hospitals maintain surge capacity for physical illness, mental health systems must anticipate surges of emotional distress. A reserve corps of counselors, psychologists, social workers, and crisis responders can be trained to mobilize during emergencies. Partnerships with universities, nonprofits, and religious organizations can create distributed networks of support that remain functional even when formal institutions falter.

What emerges is a vision of mental health as a pillar of national resilience. A psychologically fortified population is less vulnerable to manipulation, less prone to panic, and more capable of acting collectively. Emotional stability becomes a strategic asset, enabling societies to endure hardship without fracturing. Fear may spread quickly, but so can reassurance—if the channels of support are already in place.

In the crises to come, whether viral, climatic, or geopolitical, emotional resilience will be as vital as vaccines, antivirals, or logistics. A society that preserves its mental health preserves its future.

The Path Forward: Rational Humanity

A rational pandemic response is not an absence of emotion—it is the discipline to act despite emotion. It means grounding every decision in data, every policy in compassion, and every message in truth.

Science without empathy becomes technocracy; empathy without science becomes chaos. The future demands both.

If humanity learns to communicate calmly, act intelligently, and care collectively, then perhaps the next pandemic will not be a tragedy but a test we finally pass. Because preparedness is not just about stockpiles and algorithms—it is about trust, reason, and the courage to stay calm when the world begins to shake.

CHAPTER 4. THE FUTURE OF SURVIVAL: FROM QUARANTINE TO QUANTUM CITIES

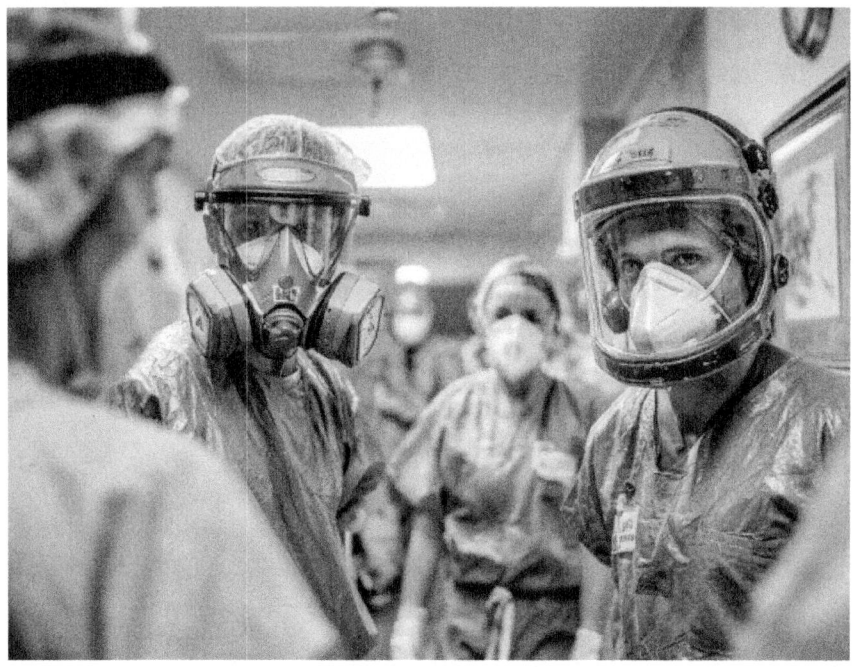

When the word *quarantine* first entered the global lexicon as something more than a historical relic, most people pictured inconvenience—a brief pause, a necessary nuisance. Few imagined it would become a worldwide experiment in isolation, testing not only the limits of our healthcare systems but the architecture of our daily lives. Yet, if the pandemic revealed anything, it was that the quality of quarantine determines the quality of human endurance.

Locking people in their homes without comfort, structure, or support was a recipe for unrest. Isolation without infrastructure breeds despair. To make quarantine both humane and effective, we must reimagine it—not as confinement, but as *protected living*.

The Architecture of Quarantine

Effective quarantine begins with logistics, not fear. People must be able to isolate without losing access to the essentials of life. Food, medicine, and daily goods must flow smoothly to those in isolation. During the pandemic, countless individuals risked infection simply to buy groceries. That risk is neither noble nor necessary.

The solution lies in a robust system of contactless delivery—drones, autonomous vehicles, and neighborhood distribution hubs that supply quarantined citizens swiftly and safely. Elderly individuals and people with disabilities, often the most vulnerable, should receive prioritized support through dedicated services. A humane society measures its progress not by the strength of its lockdowns, but by the dignity it affords its most fragile members.

Equally important is the living environment. Quarantine housing must meet both physical and psychological needs. A clean, well-equipped, and connected home is not a luxury—it's a public health measure. Internet access, for instance, has become as essential as running water. It provides not only work continuity but emotional lifelines—video calls, online therapy, entertainment, and education. Isolation, when cushioned by digital connection, becomes bearable.

Quarantine succeeds only when it becomes a system, not a slogan. The failures of 2020 revealed that most nations treated isolation as an abstract command rather than an engineered process. Houses were assumed to be safe; they were not. Supply chains were assumed to be stable; they broke. Citizens were assumed to be self-sufficient; millions were not. The result was a form of quarantine that existed on paper but collapsed in practice, forcing people into impossible choices between public safety and personal survival.

True quarantine architecture begins with anticipating human needs, not policing human behavior. Food, medication refills, sanitation supplies, and household essentials must arrive automatically once a person enters isolation. A national logistical network—integrating drones for rapid local deliveries, autonomous vehicles for bulk transport, and micro-hubs for neighborhood distribution—would convert isolation from a burden into a supported state of temporary retreat. This model mirrors military supply chains: soldiers do not leave their posts to find food; the system brings sustenance to them. The same principle must guide public health.

Specialized support for the most vulnerable transforms quarantine from coercion into care. Elderly citizens, those living alone, individuals with disabilities, and those with chronic illnesses require proactive contact and priority delivery systems—not as charity, but as infrastructure. Automated welfare checks, telemedicine integration, and daily status reporting protect those most at risk from the secondary harms of isolation: neglect, malnutrition, dehydration, untreated illness, or mental deterioration. A compassionate quarantine system is a mirror of a compassionate civilization.

Housing, too, must be reimagined. Dense urban apartments without ventilation, lacking private space, or shared by multiple generations become pressure chambers rather than protective environments. Future readiness demands the development of quarantine-capable housing units—spaces with proper airflow, sanitation facilities, and digital connectivity—designed not as emergency shelters but as standard elements of modern architecture. Even temporary modular dwellings can serve as overflow quarantine spaces when households are too crowded for safe isolation. These structures should be deployable as readily as mobile hospitals.

Connectivity is not a luxury but a lifeline. Digital access prevents the psychological collapse that so often accompanies isolation. It allows quarantined individuals to maintain their work, continue their education, participate in therapy, attend community events, and remain tethered to friends and family. A society that denies digital access denies emotional survival. Universal broadband must therefore be recognized as a public health asset, as essential as electricity or refrigeration.

The ethical dimension of quarantine lies in reciprocity. When the state asks individuals to isolate for the collective good, it must guarantee their welfare in return. Quarantine without support is abandonment disguised as policy. Quarantine with comprehensive care becomes a civic partnership: citizens fulfill their responsibility to protect others, and society fulfills its responsibility to protect them.

In the next pandemic, the measure of our progress will not be how quickly we can enforce isolation, but how effectively we can sustain those who undergo it. A well-designed quarantine system transforms an act of separation into an act of solidarity. It ensures that no one faces danger alone and that collective safety does not require individual sacrifice beyond necessity.

Mind and Body in Captivity

The body, too, demands attention during isolation. Physical inactivity is the silent accomplice of disease. Even during lockdowns, opportunities for movement— guided home workouts, online yoga sessions, and meditation apps—can transform confinement into resilience. A society that encourages fitness in quarantine is one that invests in recovery before illness even begins.

Yet the greater challenge lies in mental health. Extended isolation can erode the psyche, feeding anxiety, loneliness, and depression. The antidote is accessible psychological support: hotlines, online consultations, and digital communities where empathy travels faster than despair. Governments must treat mental well-being not as an optional afterthought but as a core element of crisis response.

Finally, there is the question of economics. For those unable to work during quarantine, financial stress often becomes as dangerous as the virus itself. Income support and compensation programs are essential—because survival should not come at the cost of bankruptcy. When people are secure, they comply; when they fear destitution, they revolt.

In short, effective quarantine must protect not only bodies, but lives in their full dimension—economic, social, and emotional.

The Lifeline of Small Business

While individuals endured isolation, another organism suffered quietly but no less gravely: the small business. Cafés, workshops, stores, and startups—the living tissue of the local economy—found themselves strangled by lockdowns. For them, survival required more than goodwill; it required strategic intervention.

Supporting small business during crises is not charity—it is self-preservation. Direct financial aid in the form of subsidies or interest-free loans can keep small enterprises afloat, preserving employment and supply continuity. Tax deferrals and rate reductions give breathing space. Temporary suspension of rent obligations can prevent the domino collapse of local commerce.

But resilience isn't just about keeping doors open—it's about adaptation. Governments and banks should invest in helping small businesses transition into the digital economy: e-commerce platforms, online services, and remote customer engagement. A world forced indoors also became a world online; those who moved fastest survived.

Equally vital is fair access to public contracts. Governments can support small enterprises by reserving portions of procurement for them—whether for goods, logistics, or digital services—turning crisis spending into an engine of recovery.

And when the storm subsides, the same programs that saved businesses can help them evolve. Grants for innovation and technological modernization can transform temporary survival into long-term growth. In this sense, crisis becomes metamorphosis—the pressure that produces resilience.

Learning the Hard Lessons

Every disaster offers data; every mistake offers insight. The true failure is not error, but repetition. To prepare for the next pandemic, societies must treat the COVID-19 era as an open book of lessons written in loss.

First, we must scrutinize the effectiveness of containment measures. Which restrictions truly saved lives, and which only paralyzed economies? A targeted, data-driven approach—based on local infection patterns and healthcare capacity—can replace the blunt instrument of total lockdown. Future crises demand surgical precision, not panic-driven overreach.

Second, healthcare systems must undergo a cold audit of readiness. Staffing shortages, equipment scarcities, and fractured coordination revealed themselves as chronic conditions long before the virus arrived. Building reserve hospitals, cross-regional medical alliances, and rapid deployment teams can close these gaps before the next wave hits.

Third, the logistics of testing and vaccination must evolve. The world needs protocols that can deploy diagnostics and vaccines at lightning speed. Streamlined regulation, automation, and AI-assisted logistics will shorten the fatal lag between discovery and distribution.

Finally, the social contract itself must be rewritten. Economic safety nets must be automatic, not improvised. Support for individuals and small businesses should trigger the moment crisis indicators appear—not weeks or months later. A truly prepared society reacts faster than fear can spread.

The Great Dispersion: Rethinking the City

And now we arrive at the most radical of conclusions—a vision that rewrites the geography of civilization itself. For centuries, humanity has celebrated its cities as triumphs of progress. Towers, traffic, and teeming millions were seen as signs of success. Then came the virus, and the skyscrapers turned into cages.

What if the greatest act of progress is not to build *up*, but to spread *out*?

Urban disintegration—the strategic dispersal of

populations into modular, autonomous dwellings—might be the boldest pandemic prevention plan ever conceived. Imagine millions no longer clustered in suffocating megacities, but living freely in intelligent, self-sustaining homes scattered across the landscape.

The modular home—like the *Boxabl*—embodies this revolution. Delivered folded on a truck and unfolded into a fully functional dwelling, it transforms housing from a stationary fortress into a mobile ecosystem. It's housing that thinks like a machine: adaptable, scalable, and recyclable.

Modern society continues to tolerate unnecessary crowding not because it is needed, but because it is inherited from an earlier industrial logic that no longer serves any functional purpose. The daily concentration of millions of people in dense cores—offices, transport nodes, commercial towers—persists out of habit rather than necessity. Digital infrastructure, remote work, autonomous delivery systems, and modular housing have already rendered much of this physical convergence obsolete. When people no longer depend on centralized buildings for their livelihoods, and when essential services can be delivered without human clustering, the very idea of mass physical concentration becomes an anachronism. In such a world, clusters do not exist as emergency structures designed only for pandemics; they exist because they reflect a more efficient, humane, and technologically aligned way of living.

This makes quarantine not a dramatic interruption of life, but a simple operational adjustment. A cluster is already a self-contained micro-community whose routine does not depend on continuous physical interchange with distant centers of population. When an infection arises, sealing the cluster does not disrupt the broader society, because the cluster was never designed as a porous node in a dense urban web. Isolation becomes a temporary narrowing of contacts, not a suspension of economic or social functioning. The population does not need to be relocated, confined, or deprived of access to goods, because logistics flow through autonomous channels that do not require human presence. In effect, the cluster model turns quarantine from a coercive, civilization-wide trauma into a routine administrative measure—targeted, proportionate, and entirely compatible with normal life.

The deeper point is that once crowding is removed from the structure of daily life, quarantine ceases to be a blunt instrument. It becomes the equivalent of circuit-breaking in an electrical grid: precise, localized, and quickly reversible. A society built from clusters can isolate exactly what must be isolated while allowing the rest to remain fully functional. This is not simply better pandemic management; it is a more rational design for human living overall. The elimination of unnecessary crowding makes societies healthier, calmer, and more resilient—and as a natural consequence, far easier to protect when biological threats do emerge.

Modular Civilization

Why endure urban chaos when one can live surrounded by nature, connected through global satellite internet, and free from the noise of neighbors? In modular living, the commute vanishes, pollution dwindles, and property becomes portable. Cities could shrink into cultural and administrative hubs, while daily life flourishes across the countryside.

The distinction between centralized and distributed living is not a simplistic opposition but a historical turning point. Crowding was once a necessity of industrial civilization: factories required workers to gather, schools required students to be present, commerce required physical markets, and culture required mass venues. None of this is true anymore. Digital infrastructure has eliminated every practical reason for millions of people to occupy the same few square miles. What remains of centralization today is not function but inertia. Once the technological need for crowding disappears, its social costs—crime, violence, stress, anonymity, noise, and systemic vulnerability—stand naked without justification. Distributed, cluster-based living is not an ideological alternative to the city; it is simply the first form of settlement aligned with the realities of the twenty-first century, in which large human aggregations are unnecessary for work, education, logistics, culture, or governance. When concentration is no longer required, its risks become intolerable. Clusters do not replace cities; they replace the need to crowd.

Urban dispersion addresses more than health. It solves housing inflation, transportation congestion, and environmental degradation. The further we move from the crowded centers, the cheaper land becomes—and the freer people are.

The proposal for dispersed modular clusters is not a spatial solution to a non-spatial problem. It is the architectural expression of a deeper technological shift: the internetization of work, culture, science, and social exchange. When most employment is digital, when education is platform-based, when research is collaborative across borders, and when culture circulates through global networks rather than physical venues, density is no longer the engine of productivity. In such a world, dispersion does not undermine economic or intellectual life—it liberates it from the bottlenecks of geography. The modular cluster is not a retreat from civilization but its modernization: a form of living designed for a society whose creative, cultural, and economic functions already occur online. The question is not how to replicate the old city, but why we continue forcing twenty-first-century life into nineteenth-century spatial constraints.

Autonomous homes powered by solar panels, equipped with rainwater filtration and composting systems, can function entirely off-grid. Smart batteries and AI energy management will ensure sustainability. With no dependence on centralized utilities, every home becomes a fortress of independence—a private biosphere immune to blackouts and breakdowns.

The economic burden of the transition is far lower than critics assume. The model does not dismantle existing structures but allows new ones to grow where demand naturally appears. It is not a revolution against industry but an adjustment of incentives that makes outdated forms of settlement less attractive and modular clusters more viable. The costs are distributed over time, absorbed by voluntary migration patterns, and supported by a microtransaction tax capable of generating unprecedented state revenues without raising the burden on individuals or businesses. The future is not built by demolishing the old but by allowing the new to outcompete it.

And there's humor in the logic: in a dispersed world, even global catastrophes lose their sting. Nuclear strike? You're miles from anyone. Earthquake? Your modular house can flex, or you can just move it. Flood? Relocate uphill. Alien invasion? Good luck finding you.

The Road Network as a Civilization Framework

Imagine transforming the existing road network into the skeleton of a new civilization. The United States alone has roughly 6.6 million kilometers of roads—enough to host nearly two billion people in modular homes, assuming modest spacing.

Instead of vertical megacities, we could have horizontal civilizations: communities stretched like pearls along highways and country roads, each home self-sufficient, each cluster connected by intelligent logistics. Drones would deliver goods from central hubs to scattered homes, guided by artificial intelligence optimizing routes by weather, terrain, and demand.

Drones are not speculative tools awaiting maturity; they are already operating in the harshest environments humans have ever engineered. A system that can identify and strike a moving armored vehicle under electronic interference is more than capable of delivering medication to a stationary home along a known route. War has already performed the stress test that peaceful logistics will never require. The question, therefore, is not technological readiness but civilizational willingness. The infrastructure exists; only the mindset lags behind.

Each hub would act as a nerve center—receiving supplies, managing energy flow, and maintaining communication. The infrastructure already exists; it only requires a new mindset. With AI coordination, delivery drones could bring groceries, medications, or even replacement home modules directly to one's door—no traffic jams, no contagion, no queues.

Within a decade, this isn't science fiction—it's simply unimplemented science.

Preparing for the Unthinkable

Urban downsizing and autonomous housing are not just conveniences—they are shields against apocalypse. Rising sea levels? Move inland. Nuclear war? Fewer concentrated targets. Asteroid impact? Dispersal means survival. Earthquake? Your home flexes, not collapses.

The great irony of modern civilization is that we've built ourselves into targets—economic, environmental, and existential. By scattering intelligently, we become harder to destroy and easier to sustain. A decentralized humanity is a resilient humanity.

In this light, modular living is not an eccentric architectural fantasy but the logical next stage of human adaptation. It represents independence, flexibility, and survival—the very qualities that evolution itself rewards.

Toward a Civilized Resilience

The pandemic was not merely a health crisis; it was a stress test of civilization. It showed us which systems bend and which break. The lesson, now painfully clear, is that survival in the modern world depends on adaptability.

Improving quarantine conditions, supporting local economies, learning from failure, and reshaping how and where we live—these are not separate initiatives but interconnected facets of a single philosophy: *resilient living*.

The future will belong to those who prepare not by hoarding, but by evolving. Those who understand that the true antidote to crisis is not control, but creativity.

Because pandemics, wars, and disasters will come again. The question is not *if*—it's *how ready we'll be when they do*.

Afterword. Lessons from the Plague: Between Fear and Freedom

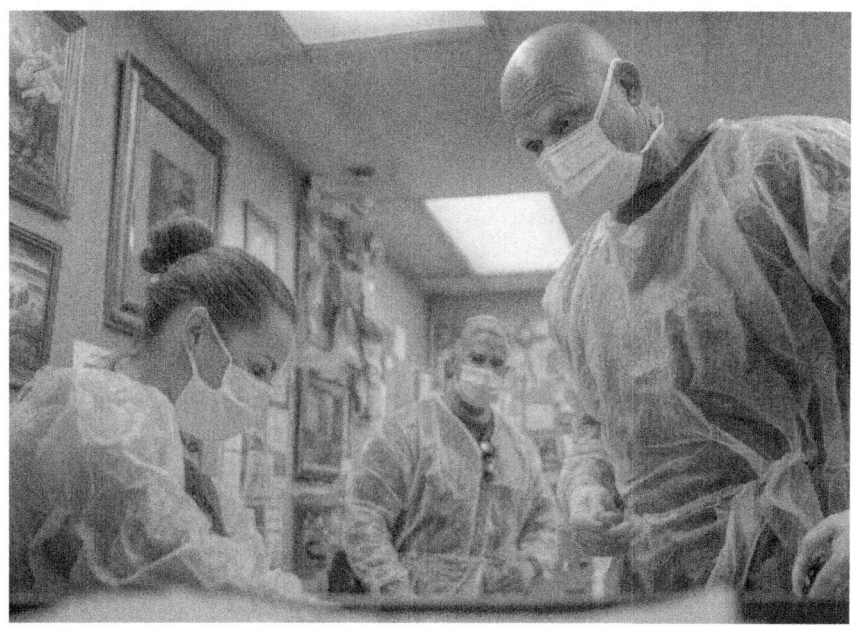

As the dust of the pandemic finally settles and cities once again hum with life, I find myself haunted by a question that refuses to fade: *What have we actually learned from all this?*

We endured years of fear, control, isolation, and loss. The world we knew dissolved almost overnight—streets emptied, faces vanished behind masks, human contact was replaced by screens. Now, as we return to something resembling normality, I can't help but wonder whether we have truly understood what happened to us, or whether we've merely chosen to forget.

The coronavirus pandemic was more than a health crisis. It was a mirror, brutally honest and unflattering, reflecting not just the weakness of our bodies but the fragility of our societies, our institutions, and our values. The virus tested our science, yes—but it tested our humanity even more.

The Logic of Survival

At its core, the idea of downsizing civilization—of replacing dense cities with autonomous, modular homes—represents more than a technological dream. It's a philosophy of resilience. By dispersing populations, decentralizing resources, and embracing self-sufficiency, humanity could finally become less fragile, less dependent, less vulnerable.

In such a system, pandemics, wars, and natural disasters lose much of their destructive potential. A modular civilization can move, adapt, and survive. Every home could generate its own energy, recycle its own water, and function as a node in a global network of intelligent, sustainable living.

Remote work, long dismissed as a niche convenience, proved during the pandemic that physical proximity is often an outdated relic. Many professions operate perfectly well from afar. Reducing unnecessary contact not only improves public safety but enhances productivity, cuts costs, and spares the environment.

The great irony of the modern age is that technology liberated us long ago—but we kept pretending we were still chained to offices and cities. The pandemic shattered that illusion. The future belongs to the flexible—the societies that can disperse without disconnecting.

The Rise of the Machines (That Serve Humanity)

If people are to live farther apart, logistics must become smarter. The delivery of goods, services, and even medical care will depend on precision and intelligence. Artificial intelligence and machine learning will become the nervous system of this new world—analyzing data, predicting needs, optimizing routes, and ensuring that no one is too remote to be reached.

AI-driven logistics could make long-distance delivery faster than local shopping ever was. Drones and automated vehicles will form an invisible ballet in the sky and on the roads, ensuring contactless, efficient, and safe distribution. The pandemic hinted at this future; the next crisis will demand it.

The same applies to healthcare. Remote diagnostics, AI-assisted consultations, and telemedicine can ensure that even isolated individuals receive care equal to that of major hospitals. In a dispersed civilization, distance becomes irrelevant; data bridges the gap.

Freedom and Its Discontents

But for all the technological promise, one cannot ignore the darker legacy of the pandemic: the ease with which fear devoured freedom.

Personal liberties—the cornerstone of any civilized society—were suspended, sometimes brutally, under the banner of safety. Curfews, travel bans, forced isolation, digital surveillance—measures that once belonged to dystopian fiction became everyday life. What began as public health policy often morphed into bureaucratic domination, stripped of logic or proportion.

No one denies that emergency measures were needed in the early stages. Quarantine, after all, is as old as plague itself. But as the virus spread and evolved, many restrictions remained long after they ceased to make sense. The result was an avalanche of economic destruction, social alienation, and psychological collapse.

The worst sin was not the fear—it was the *hypocrisy*. Governments, corporations, and institutions exploited the crisis for control, profit, and political theater. Behind every "stay safe" slogan lurked a committee calculating advantage. Humanity's collective terror became a market commodity and a political weapon.

And so, in the name of protection, freedom was sold cheaply, and dignity became expendable.

The Question of Origins

There is little doubt, in my view, that the pandemic began not in the chaotic swirl of nature but in the sterile corridors of a laboratory. The circumstantial evidence is overwhelming. Few cities in the world host facilities engaged in such virological research, and it is no coincidence that the outbreak began precisely there. Whether this was an accident or something more deliberate may never matter as much as what followed—the manipulation, the secrecy, the opportunism.

The discussion of viral origins in this book is not meant as a definitive scientific adjudication between competing hypotheses. Whether a pathogen emerges from wildlife spillover, laboratory accidents, or ecological disturbance, the practical implications for preparedness are the same: societies must be structurally resilient to biological uncertainty from any source. The point is not to promote a political narrative but to underscore a systemic vulnerability that transcends the natural-versus-artificial dichotomy. Modern science acknowledges multiple plausible pathways for viral emergence, and responsible policy does not depend on choosing one but on building systems robust to all. The argument is therefore not causal speculation—it is a call for architectural readiness regardless of origin.

What should have been a scientific tragedy became a geopolitical performance. Instead of transparency, we got propaganda. Instead of collaboration, we got rivalry. Humanity was fighting a virus—and each other.

The deeper tragedy of the origin debate is not which hypothesis is ultimately correct, but how quickly the search for truth dissolved into a contest of narratives. Whether the first breach occurred in a marketplace, through zoonotic transfer, or in a laboratory setting—accidental or otherwise—the response should have been the same: immediate transparency, immediate cooperation, immediate mobilization of global expertise. Instead, the world was thrust into a fog of competing explanations, each shaped less by science than by political self-interest.

The scientific community itself was caught between incomplete data and an atmosphere of geopolitical pressure. Early analyses of the viral genome did not conclusively favor either scenario. Natural spillover, a historically common pathway for emerging pathogens, remained plausible. So did laboratory involvement, given the proximity of high-level virological institutes and the well-documented global history of laboratory leaks involving other pathogens. What made clarity impossible was not biology but obstruction. Critical records, early case data, and sample repositories were restricted or sanitized before independent investigators could access them. This manufactured ambiguity became a breeding ground for speculation, suspicion, and public distrust.

The real failure was not the origin—it was the reaction to uncertainty. In a functioning global system, absence of evidence triggers cooperation; in our world, it triggered defensiveness. Governments treated the question as a battlefield for prestige rather than a matter of planetary security. Nations accused each other, deflected responsibility, or weaponized the ambiguity to advance unrelated agendas. Instead of a unified scientific inquiry, humanity received a geopolitical circus.

This fragmentation had consequences beyond narrative. The lack of transparent early information delayed international recognition of the outbreak's severity. Containment windows closed. Borders remained open when they should have narrowed and narrowed when they no longer mattered. Early genomic sequences were released reluctantly or incompletely, slowing the development of diagnostics and early prototypes of vaccines. Public trust eroded as contradictory statements accumulated. The world was left fighting not only a pathogen but a shadow war of secrecy and doubt.

The lesson for the future is not to fixate on which origin theory one prefers but to recognize that **origin transparency is a non-negotiable duty of civilization**. Any high-risk virological research must be governed by international oversight, mandatory disclosure protocols, and independent auditing. Any outbreak—anywhere— must trigger automatic release of full epidemiological data to global systems. No nation has the right to conceal threat information that endangers the entire species. Pathogens do not respect borders; therefore, neither can knowledge.

Humanity's vulnerability emerges not from how pandemics begin but from how truth is handled in their first days. Secrecy is itself a biological accelerant. Rivalry is a form of epidemiological sabotage. A civilization that cannot share information cannot protect itself. The question of origins will matter less in hindsight than whether our species learns to create a world where origins, whatever they may be, can never be hidden again.

The Mask and the Theater

Masks, vaccines, lockdowns—each became less a medical measure and more a political symbol. The science of prevention was drowned in the politics of compliance.

Masks, for example, were useful not because they stopped the virus itself, but because they reduced the spread of infected droplets. Yet they also became emblems—of virtue to some, oppression to others. Mandates enforced by threat of penalty crossed the line from recommendation into coercion.

Vaccines, too, lost their scientific innocence, becoming subjects of corporate monopoly and state control. Their initial success against early strains of the virus was undeniable—but as mutations appeared, efficacy fell, and faith along with it. The world would have done better to invest equally in antiviral drugs, like Paxlovid, which directly attack viral replication and remain effective regardless of mutation.

Instead, pharmaceutical giants pursued profits while governments pursued political redemption. Humanity got neither immunity nor wisdom.

The Cost of Overreach

The tragedy of the pandemic lies in its imbalance. The obsession with controlling the virus overshadowed everything else. Businesses collapsed, mental health eroded, and other medical conditions went untreated. Cancer screenings halted, heart patients missed surgeries, and suicide rates climbed. The "cure" often inflicted wounds deeper than the disease.

What was needed was nuance—a flexible, targeted approach rather than blanket decrees. Instead of locking down entire nations, we could have protected the elderly and chronically ill, provided focused support to vulnerable populations, and kept the rest of society functioning.

Testing and contact tracing, used effectively in places like South Korea and Taiwan, could have contained outbreaks without paralyzing economies. Public education, not coercion, should have been the guiding principle. When people understand the *why*, they are more willing to accept the *what*.

But the arrogance of authority replaced reason with decree, and science with spectacle.

Toward a Rational Humanity

From all this chaos, one truth emerges: a civilized society must never again trade liberty for the illusion of safety. True preparedness lies not in control, but in competence.

To face the future, we need systems that learn and adapt:

- **A unified global healthcare network** that shares data instantly and transparently.

- **AI-driven logistics and telemedicine**, ensuring access to care and supplies everywhere.

- **Flexible labor systems** that embrace remote work, preserving both productivity and safety.

- **Targeted, data-based crisis measures**, instead of indiscriminate restrictions.

- **Ongoing psychological and economic support programs**, protecting people from despair as much as disease.

Preparedness is not about fortifying walls—it's about connecting minds.

After the Silence

Now, as the masks come off and laughter returns to the streets, the question remains: *Was it worth it?*

We've seen the human spirit buckle under fear, and

freedom traded for the comfort of obedience. We've witnessed the grotesque spectacle of politicians and corporations turning catastrophe into currency. The twenty-first-century plague exposed not only the weakness of our immune systems, but the hollowness of our moral ones.

The opportunity to grow wiser and stronger was there— and we squandered it. Instead of unity, we chose division. Instead of reflection, distraction. Instead of reform, denial.

And so, here we are—alive, perhaps, but unchanged. The next crisis will come, as it always does. And when it does, I fear that this book, like so many warnings before it, will simply become another voice crying in the wilderness.

Still, one must write. One must hope. Because even if humanity refuses to learn, the act of remembering is, in itself, a form of resistance.

BIBLIOGRAPHY

Abrams, E. M., & Szefler, S. J. (2020). COVID-19 and the impact of social determinants of health. *The Lancet Respiratory Medicine*, 8, 659–661.

Alexander, C., Ishikawa, S., & Silverstein, M. (1977). *A pattern language: Towns, buildings, construction.* Oxford University Press.

Anderson, R. M., Heesterbeek, H., Klinkenberg, D., & Hollingsworth, T. D. (2020). How will country-based mitigation measures influence the course of the COVID-19 epidemic? *The Lancet*, 395, 931–934.

Apple Inc., & Google LLC. (2020). *Exposure Notification: Bluetooth specification and cryptography.*

Ardila, D., et al. (2019). End-to-end lung cancer screening with three-dimensional deep learning on low-dose chest CT. *Nature Medicine*, 25, 954–961.

Arendt, H. (1958). *The human condition.* University of Chicago Press.

Baden, L. R., et al. (2021). Efficacy and safety of the mRNA-1273 SARS-CoV-2 vaccine. *New England Journal of Medicine*, 384, 403–416.

Bar-On, Y. M., et al. (2021). Protection of BNT162b2 vaccine booster against Covid-19 in Israel. *New England Journal of Medicine*, 385, 1393–1400.

Bavel, J. J. V., et al. (2020). Using social and behavioural science to support COVID-19 pandemic response. *Nature Human Behaviour*, 4, 460–471.

Beigel, J. H., et al. (2020). Remdesivir for the treatment of Covid-19 — Final report. *New England Journal of Medicine*, 383, 1813–1826.

Christakis, N. A. (2020). *Apollo's Arrow: The profound and enduring impact of coronavirus on the way we live*. Little, Brown.

Dagan, N., et al. (2021). BNT162b2 mRNA Covid-19 vaccine in a nationwide mass vaccination setting. *New England Journal of Medicine*, 384, 1412–1423.

Diamond, J. (2005). *Collapse: How societies choose to fail or succeed*. Viking.

Dong, E., Du, H., & Gardner, L. (2020). An interactive web-based dashboard to track COVID-19 in real time. *The Lancet Infectious Diseases*, 20, 533–534.

Emanuel, E. J., et al. (2020). Fair allocation of scarce medical resources in the time of Covid-19. *New England Journal of Medicine*, 382, 2049–2055.

European Centre for Disease Prevention and Control. (2020). *Guidance for health system preparedness for COVID-19*.

Fauci, A. S., Lane, H. C., & Redfield, R. R. (2020). Covid-19 — Navigating the uncharted. *New England Journal of Medicine*, 382, 1268–1269.

Ferguson, N. M., et al. (2020). *Impact of non-pharmaceutical interventions (NPIs) to reduce COVID-19 mortality and healthcare demand* (Report 9). Imperial College London.

Flaxman, S., et al. (2020). Estimating the effects of non-pharmaceutical interventions on COVID-19 in Europe. *Nature, 584*, 257–261.

Foucault, M. (1977). *Discipline and punish: The birth of the prison.* Pantheon.

Gawande, A. (2010). *The checklist manifesto.* Metropolitan Books.

Giddens, A. (1999). *Runaway world: How globalization is reshaping our lives.* Profile Books.

Greenhalgh, T., et al. (2021). Ten scientific reasons in support of airborne transmission of SARS-CoV-2. *The Lancet, 397*, 1603–1605.

Habermas, J. (1984). *The theory of communicative action* (Vol. 1). Beacon Press.

Hamidi, S., Sabouri, S., & Ewing, R. (2020). Does density aggravate the COVID-19 pandemic? *Journal of the American Planning Association, 86*, 495–509.

Hammond, J., et al. (2022). Oral nirmatrelvir for high-risk, nonhospitalized adults with Covid-19. *New England Journal of Medicine, 386*, 1397–1408.

He, X., et al. (2020). Temporal dynamics in viral shedding and transmissibility of COVID-19. *Nature Medicine, 26*, 672–675.

Hellewell, J., et al. (2020). Feasibility of controlling COVID-19 outbreaks by isolation of cases and contacts. *The Lancet Global Health*, 8, e488–e496.

Institute of Medicine. (2012). *Crisis standards of care: A systems framework for catastrophic disaster response.* National Academies Press.

Ioannidis, J. P. A. (2005). Why most published research findings are false. *PLoS Medicine*, 2, e124.

Jayk Bernal, A., et al. (2022). Molnupiravir for oral treatment of Covid-19 in nonhospitalized patients. *New England Journal of Medicine*, 386, 509–520.

Kahneman, D. (2011). *Thinking, fast and slow.* Farrar, Straus and Giroux.

Keesara, S., Jonas, A., & Schulman, K. (2020). Covid-19 and health care's digital revolution. *New England Journal of Medicine*, 382, e82.

Kissler, S. M., Tedijanto, C., Goldstein, E., Grad, Y. H., & Lipsitch, M. (2020). Projecting the transmission dynamics of SARS-CoV-2 through the postpandemic period. *Science*, 368, 860–868.

Li, R., et al. (2020). Substantial undocumented infection facilitates the rapid dissemination of novel coronavirus (SARS-CoV-2). *Science*, 368, 489–493.

Lopez Bernal, J., et al. (2021). Effectiveness of Covid-19 vaccines against the B.1.617.2 (Delta) variant. *New England Journal of Medicine*, 385, 585–594.

Lurie, N., Saville, M., Hatchett, R., & Halton, J. (2020). Developing Covid-19 vaccines at pandemic speed. *New England Journal of Medicine*, 382, 1969–1973.

Mandel, J. C., et al. (2016). SMART on FHIR: A standards-based, interoperable apps platform for electronic health records. *Journal of the American Medical Informatics Association*, 23, 899–908.

McNeill, W. H. (1976). *Plagues and peoples*. Anchor.

Mishra, T., et al. (2020). Early detection of COVID-19 using smartwatch data. *NPJ Digital Medicine*, 3, 156.

Morawska, L., & Milton, D. K. (2020). It is time to address airborne transmission of COVID-19. *Clinical Infectious Diseases*, 71, 2311–2313.

Morens, D. M., Folkers, G. K., & Fauci, A. S. (2009). The challenge of emerging and re-emerging infectious diseases. *New England Journal of Medicine*, 360, 2151–2153.

National Academies of Sciences, Engineering, and Medicine. (2020). *Rapid expert consultation on the possibility of bioaerosol spread of SARS-CoV-2*. National Academies Press.

National Academies of Sciences, Engineering, and Medicine. (2022). *Lessons from the COVID-19 pandemic to improve public health preparedness*. National Academies Press.

National Audit Office. (2020). *The government's approach to test and trace in England — Interim report*.

Office of the Auditor General of Canada. (2021). *Report 8: Pandemic preparedness, surveillance, and border control measures.*

Osterholm, M. T., & Olshaker, M. (2017). *Deadliest enemy: Our war against killer germs.* Little, Brown.

Polack, F. P., et al. (2020). Safety and efficacy of the BNT162b2 mRNA Covid-19 vaccine. *New England Journal of Medicine,* 383, 2603–2615.

Porter, M. E. (2010). What is value in health care? *New England Journal of Medicine,* 363, 2477–2481.

Prather, K. A., Marr, L. C., Schooley, R. T., McDiarmid, M. A., Wilson, M. E., & Milton, D. K. (2020). Airborne transmission of SARS-CoV-2. *Science,* 370, 303–304.

Rosenbaum, L. (2020). Facing Covid-19 in Italy — Ethics, logistics, and therapeutics on the front line. *New England Journal of Medicine,* 382, 1873–1875.

Sanmarchi, F., et al. (2021). Exploring the gap between excess mortality and COVID-19 deaths in Italy. *BMC Public Health,* 21, 530.

Sen, A. (1999). *Development as freedom.* Alfred A. Knopf.

Shu, Y., & McCauley, J. (2017). GISAID: Global initiative on sharing all influenza data — From vision to reality. *Eurosurveillance,* 22, 30494.

Taleb, N. N. (2010). *The Black Swan: The impact of the highly improbable* (2nd ed.). Random House.

Tian, H., et al. (2020). An investigation of transmission control measures during the first 50 days of the COVID-19 epidemic in

China. *Science*, 368, 638–642.

Topol, E. J. (2019). High-performance medicine: The convergence of human and artificial intelligence. *Nature Medicine*, 25, 44–56.

Tufte, E. R. (2001). *The visual display of quantitative information* (2nd ed.). Graphics Press.

United Nations Children's Fund. (2021). *Unmanned aircraft systems (UAS) in immunization: A landscape analysis*. UNICEF.

Voysey, M., et al. (2021). Safety and efficacy of the ChAdOx1 nCoV-19 vaccine (AZD1222). *The Lancet*, 397, 99–111.

Wang, C., Horby, P. W., Hayden, F. G., & Gao, G. F. (2020). A novel coronavirus outbreak of global health concern. *The Lancet*, 395, 470–473.

World Health Organization. (2020). *COVID-19 strategic preparedness and response plan*. WHO.

World Health Organization. (2020). *Operational considerations for case management of COVID-19 in health facility and community*. WHO.

Zarocostas, N. (2020). How to fight an infodemic. *The Lancet*, 395, 676.

Printed in Dunstable, United Kingdom

73599498R00127